The CBD COOKBOOK *for* BEGINNERS

100 Simple and Delicious Recipes Using CBD

MARY J. WHITE

Houghton Mifflin Harcourt · Boston · New York · 2019

Copyright © 2019 by Houghton Mifflin Harcourt Publishing Company

Interior text by Mary J. White

Photography by Valerie McKinley

For information about permission to reproduce selections from this book, write to trade.permissions@hmhco.com or to Permissions, Houghton Mifflin Harcourt Publishing Company, 3 Park Avenue, 19th Floor, New York, New York 10016.

hmhbooks.com

Library of Congress Cataloging-in-Publication Data

ISBN 978-0-358-34363-9 (pbk)

ISBN 978-0-358-35337-9 (ebk)

Book design by Tai Blanche

1 2331 19

Printed in the United States of America

4500779089

This book is dedicated to my guys Colin and Aaron, the best food testers anyone could ask for.

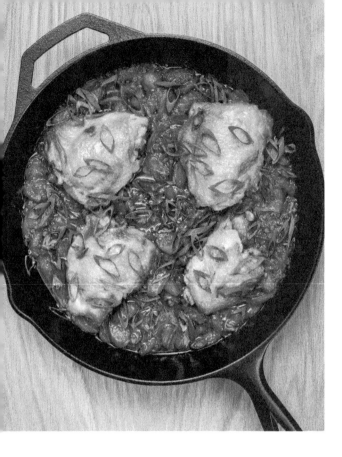

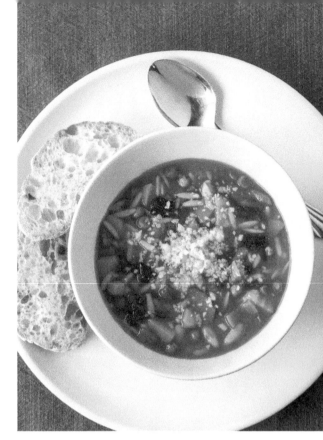

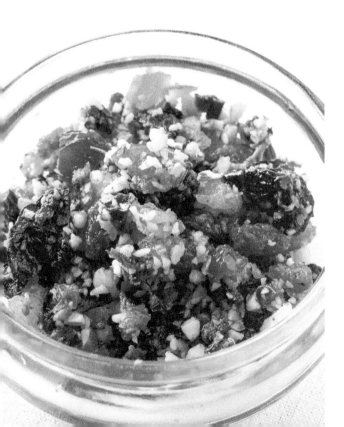

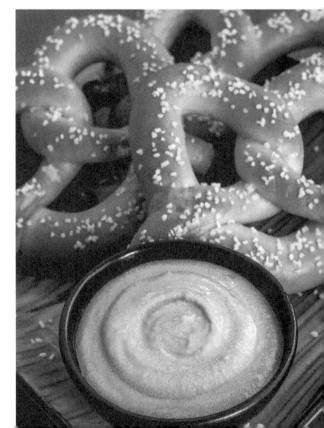

CONTENTS

INTRODUCTION

IF YOU'RE READING THIS COOKBOOK, FIRST OF ALL, THANK YOU! I'VE BEEN TEACHING HOW TO COOK WITH CANNABIS FOR YEARS NOW, AND HELPING PEOPLE FEEL BETTER IS ONE OF THE GREAT joys in my life. A few years ago I was suffering with chronic pain and taking a lot of pills for it, but I wasn't getting better. I tried a medicated cookie and was astonished at the relief I felt. I immediately started to learn all I could about medical cannabis and started teaching cooking classes. In my years of teaching cooking with cannabis, I've found many people just want to feel better—they're not interested in the recreational side of things.

In this cookbook, I'm going to show you how to use and get the benefits from CBD, that incredible compound found in *Cannabis ruderalis*, or hemp. CBD is just one of the many beneficial compounds in cannabis. I'll also share resources on how and where to buy your hemp at the end of this book.

Before we get all nervous about the word "cannabis," let's clarify. There are three primary types of cannabis: *Cannabis sativa*, *Cannabis indica*, and *Cannabis ruderalis*. If you visit a dispensary, you'll see countless hybrids—combinations of different strains with all kinds of effects—but for this book I'll be discussing only *C. ruderalis*, or hemp, as that's where your CBD will be coming from. While *C. sativa* and *C. indica* both contain more than 100 active cannabinoids, including CBD and varying amounts of THC, or delta-9-tetrahydrocannabinol (one of the compounds responsible for getting you "high") many people prefer CBD derived from *C. ruderalis*, because it does not produce a high. *Cannabis ruderalis*—but let's say "hemp" from here on—by definition has no more than .03% THC, which is not enough for you to get high.

Many people may be scared of cannabis, but cannabis-derived medicine is easily and happily accepted by our endocannabinoid system (neurotransmitters in our nervous system). It can go a long way in helping you feel better, whereas side effects from many pharmaceuticals can be far, far worse. We've been inundated with inaccurate messages about cannabis since the 1930s, but it is considered one of the best natural medicines in history. For millennia, humans have used cannabis for medicine, and before hemp was outlawed in the 1970s, land animals happily grazed on wild cannabis, providing us with naturally occurring cannabinoids in our food.

Because hemp as been treated as a controlled substance for decades, there hasn't been much scientific research on it. Scientists are only now starting to study the potential benefits of CBD, proper dosing, and possible interaction with other medicines. So, no one can say whether cooking with CBD will be useful as to any particular condition or for any particular person. But, here is what I've observed:

I've been making CBD oil for a while for my dear friend Molly, who has issues from type 1 diabetes. She doesn't like the feeling of being high but needed relief from associated physical challenges, including some issues with her hands. After just a couple of weeks ingesting my homemade CBD bites, her hands are fine and she finds her whole system works better. My pal Sara, who had a severe stroke a few years ago, is now walking without a cane thanks to CBD. I also make a coconut oil–based CBD extraction for our fur babies; my cat Hugo J. Treadwell gets it, as do many of my friends' overactive dogs. It really helps to calm them down. I could go on and on, but the main message is this: CBD is great natural medicine.

If you are just learning about cannabis, trying products containing CBD is a good starting point. However, you should be very aware of where your products come from. A lot of the CBD products on the market are full of pesticides and heavy metals, among other things. Hemp is a "soil cleaner," another of its wonderful properties, but that can mean your hemp might soak up unhealthy contaminants in the soil in which it grows. Look for "organic" and "grown in the U.S." if possible.

Look for "organic" and "grown in the U.S." if possible.

A note on cooking with CBD: It's important to me that these recipes are accessible, so all of the ones you'll find in this book are relatively easy, and can often be done in 30 minutes or less. Ceramic, glass, and stainless steel are your best bet for bowls, pans, and cooking vessels—aluminum or copper will react with the CBD and give you less-than-delicious results. I encourage you to play with your food and experiment, as the taste of CBD extracts can be challenging to get used to, and everyone's taste buds have different preferences. (More on this in the next chapter.)

AN IMPORTANT WORD ABOUT SAFETY AND LEGALITY

Children or pregnant or nursing women should not consume CBD or foods containing CBD. Do not give medicated foods to anyone without their knowledge. Also, it is unknown whether CBD may interact with other medicines. In addition, we recommend exercising caution if you choose to mix CBD with alcohol, including when preparing any recipes herein. The information herein does not constitute medical advice. Check with your health care provider prior to using CBD if you have questions.

As of the time of printing, hemp is legal pursuant to federal laws. However, some states classify hemp as a controlled substance (marijuana) under state law. The recipes and discussion herein do not constitute legal advice or advocate for violation of any laws.

FROM CANNABIS *to* CBD

CBD DOSAGE GUIDELINES

It's good to know how much CBD is in what you're making. However, there are a lot of variables: the quality of your hemp, your oven temperature, your preparation methods, and more. Most of us are used to Western medicine, where everything is measured in exact milligrams, but you are infusing different mediums (fats, alcohol, glycerin) with a natural plant material, so dosing needs to be approached differently. Cooking with cannabis is very much about learning what works for you. The effect you get from what you cook depends on the strain, how it was prepared, and the amount ingested, as well as other variables, so be aware and listen to your body.

Cooking with cannabis is very much about learning what works for you

Of course, one of the glorious things about using CBD is that it truly can't hurt you. Unlike opioids, CBD doesn't affect the brain stem, and there is no psychoactive effect; humans can't overdose on CBD. To give you a good general idea, **estimate 50 to 70 milligrams of CBD per gram of hemp material.**

So, if you have 1 ounce (28 grams) of hemp, after you decarboxylate it, you'll have anywhere from 1,400 to 1,960 milligrams of CBD and other cannabinoids available in that 1 ounce of hemp.

1 gram of cannabis	50 to 70 milligrams of CBD
1 ounce (28 grams) of cannabis	1,400 to 1,960 milligrams of CBD

Again, with CBD it's not about the number of milligrams, it's how you feel, so pay attention to your body. Use a little more or a little less; experimenting is half the fun!

DECARBOXYLATING CANNABIS

To get the maximum benefit from your hemp into your food, you need to *de-carboxylate*, or gently heat, the plant material first. "Decarbing" transforms the cannabinoid acids into bio-available cannabinoids, which means more CBD and other good stuff for you. After cannabis is decarbed, it's ready to be infused into butter or oil (page 7), infused into tinctures (page 10), or made into flour (see page 4) for the CBD to be truly bio-available.

There are charts available online to show you different decarboxylation times for different benefits, but when learning the basics, decarbing for 30 minutes at 225°F is a good general rule. As heat can degrade the effectiveness of cannabinoids, make sure not to bake at too high a heat or for too long.

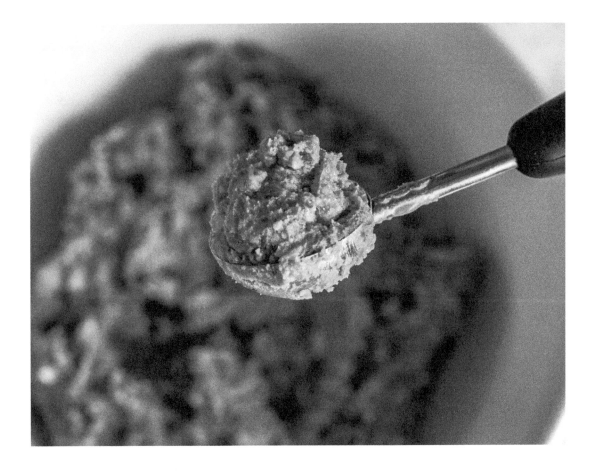

DECARBOXYLATED CANNABIS (CBD FLOUR)

Nothing could be simpler than making your own CBD flour, or finely ground decarboxylated cannabis. The key to this preparation is making sure the flour is completely dry, as mold can be an issue.

If using in place of wheat (or other) flour, the most important thing to remember is quantity: Because of the extremely strong flavor of cannabis and lack of gluten, you don't want to substitute more than one-quarter of your flour with CBD flour. Also, using CBD flour will give you a lot of CBD, so you probably won't need to use CBD butter, honey, or other CBD products in your CBD flour preparation. Play with it and see what works for you.

For plant material, cannabis "bud" is preferred, but if "shake" is all that's available, figure that the flour made from it has about half the amount of CBD as that made from bud.

Whatever you're using the decarbed hemp for, the method is the same.

Cannabis (bud is preferred, but shake will work; see Headnote)

Spread your plant material on a baking sheet and cover with foil. Place in a low oven, around 225°F, for 30 to 40 minutes. Remove from the oven, uncover, and let cool completely. It is now ready to be used to make the other products you will see in the coming pages.

A DIFFERENT DECARBING METHOD

I don't teach this in my classes because it can take several days, but if you really want to smooth out the taste and enjoy a less vegetal flavor in your CBD products, this is a good way to go. In this method, you wash out some of the chlorophyll, so your product will taste less like the lawn.

Cannabis (bud is preferred, but shake will work; see Headnote, page 4)

Big pan or sink full of warm water (not over 115°F)

Immerse your hemp in the warm water for 3 to 4 minutes. Then take it out and spread it on baking sheets to dry, away from heat and light. This should take several days. (Do not pop this in the oven to dry, as you'll have cooked off all of the CBD by the time it is dry!) Make sure it's absolutely dried out and that it hasn't grown mold.

Spread your plant material on a baking sheet and cover with foil. Place in a low oven, around 225°F, for 30 to 40 minutes. Remove from the oven, uncover, and let cool completely. It is now ready to be used to make flour (page 4) and other products.

FAT EXTRACTIONS: BUTTER AND OIL

CBD needs fat, alcohol, or glycerin to be bio-available. Butter, oil, and other fats like ghee, lard, and solid coconut oil can be infused with decarbed hemp for cooking, baking, and many other uses. A good rule when making CBD butter or CBD oil is a 1:1 ratio. In other words, 1 ounce CBD Flour (page 4) to 1 pound unsalted butter or 16 ounces of oil. Tip: Don't ever let your fat extractions boil—high temperatures will cook off the CBD. I always recommend storing these in glass in the fridge; plastic can leach out cannabinoids.

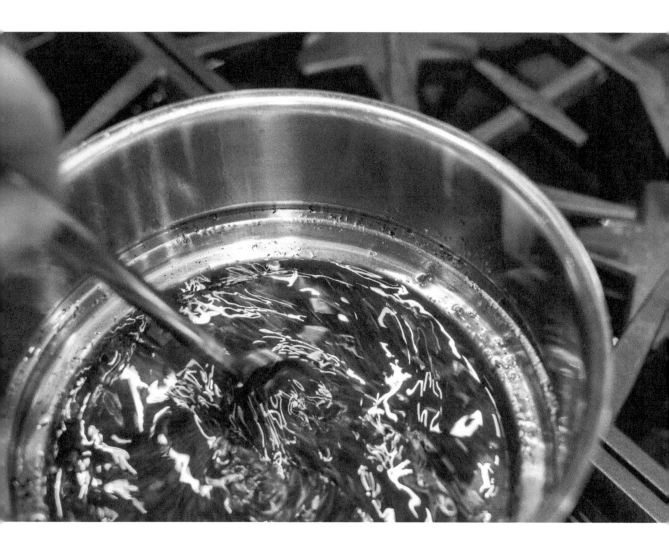

CBD BUTTER *or* OIL

It's important to cook these products gently for the best results. If the mixture gets dark brown, or if you find that your CBD products aren't working, the heat was too high and/or you cooked it too long.

1 ounce CBD Flour (page 4)

1 pound (4 sticks) unsalted butter or 16 ounces (2 cups) of olive, coconut, vegetable, or other oil of your choice

Place the flour and butter or oil in the top of a double boiler with barely simmering water below (see Note). Cook for 4 to 5 hours, making sure the mixture is barely bubbling, and stir often. Do not cook less than 4 hours or longer than 5 hours; this will affect the effectiveness of the CBD. (Check the simmering water occasionally and replenish as needed.) Strain the butter through a cheesecloth-lined sieve into a glass container and refrigerate. It is now ready to use. The butter will keep for up to a month in the fridge.

note

You can also use your slow cooker. Add 1 cup of water to the hemp mixture and cook on the low setting. Cook for 4 to 5 hours, making sure the mixture is barely bubbling, and stir often. Do not cook longer than 5 hours. Strain the butter through a cheesecloth-lined sieve into a glass container and refrigerate till the fat is solid. Lift off the fat, discard the water, and it is ready to use. Store in a glass container in the fridge for up to a month.

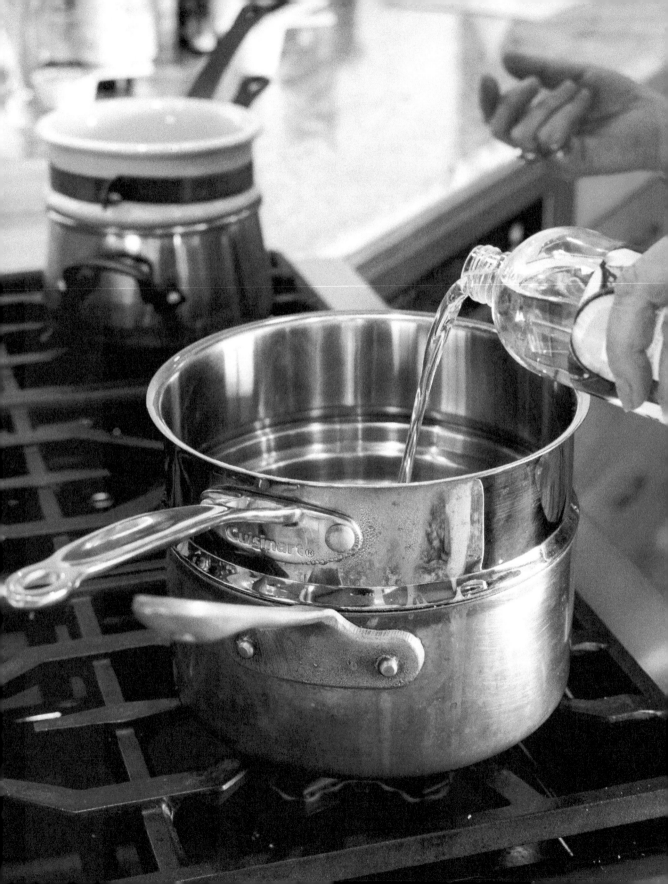

TINCTURES: GLYCERIN AND ALCOHOL

Tincture, a liquid delivery system, is an effective (and somewhat under-rated) way to get your medicine. Tinctures are usually made with strong alcohol or mild glycerin; the person using it and what it's being used for will determine the extraction method.

Taken sublingually, or absorbed under the tongue, the effects of tinctures happen faster than with other edibles, but the effects don't last quite as long, so this is often a good way to medicate. Taken in a beverage, the effects take a bit longer to kick in, as the medicine has to go through your digestive system. It is important to always store tinctures in the fridge, in glass if possible, so they remain potent. Whichever method you end up using, I'm sure you'll love the ease of use and efficiency of tinctures.

continues on next page

CBD ALCOHOL TINCTURE

Back in the day, alcohol tinctures were made by combining plant material with alcohol and letting it sit for a few weeks, but this method is much quicker. The high alcohol content in Everclear is very effective at extracting the medicinal compounds from the hemp.

It isn't recommended that you use this sublingually, as the Everclear can be intense. This alcohol CBD tincture is best used for gummies and medicating items like coffee and sugar. You can substitute regular vodka for the Everclear, but the tincture won't be as potent.

MAKES 4 OUNCES

4   ounces (½ cup) Everclear grain alcohol
4   grams CBD Flour (page 4)
2   glass jars with lids

Combine the Everclear and flour in a glass jar with a lid. Close the lid, shake, and place in the freezer for 1 hour. Take it out and shake for 3 minutes. This will shock all the medicinal compounds right out of the plant material. Strain the tincture through a strainer lined with cheesecloth into another glass jar and cover. Store in the fridge for 6 months to a year.

CBD GLYCERIN TINCTURE

This is great for anyone who doesn't want to use alcohol. The natural sweetness of the glycerin makes it more palatable to ingest, especially for pets.

MAKES 4 OUNCES

4   ounces (½ cup) vegetable glycerin
4   grams CBD Flour (page 4)
2   glass jars with lids

Combine the glycerin and flour in a glass jar with a lid. Close the lid. Line the bottom of a slow cooker with a dishcloth and fill the pot with a few inches of water, enough to cover the sides of the jar but not submerge it. (This will protect the jar from getting too hot.) Place the jar on the dishcloth in the cooker, set it to low, and let cook for 24 hours, shaking the jar a few times to ensure the mixture is combined. Strain the tincture through a strainer lined with cheesecloth into another glass jar and cover. Store in the fridge for 6 months to a year.

PANTRY *and* CONDIMENTS

CBD SUGAR

This is a great way to get CBD into your coffee, tea, or cereal—it will make your morning *way* better—or whereever else you use sugar. It's also great to take to the office to help smooth out those tough days.

MAKES 1 CUP

1 cup granulated or light brown sugar

1 to 2 tablespoons CBD Alcohol Tincture (page 10)

Preheat the oven to 200°F. Line a baking sheet with parchment paper.

In a mixing bowl, combine the sugar and the tincture. Mix with a fork to incorporate—it'll be grainy. Spread in a thin layer on the baking sheet. Bake for 30 minutes to evaporate the alcohol. Remove from the oven and let cool completely.

Press the sugar through a sieve or sifter to return it to a granulated consistency. Store in an airtight container in a dark, cool place.

CBD SALT

This is another good way to introduce some CBD into your menu. Use with abandon for happy, relaxed meals! Like the sugar recipe, this is all about the CBD tincture.

MAKES 1 CUP

1 cup fine sea salt or table salt (see Note)

1 to 3 tablespoons CBD Alcohol Tincture (page 10)

Preheat the oven to 200°F. Line a baking sheet with parchment paper.

In a bowl, combine the salt and tincture. Mix with a fork to incorporate. Spread in a thin layer on a baking sheet. Bake for 20 to 30 minutes to evaporate the alcohol. When the salt is dry and somewhat chunky, remove from the oven, break it up with the fork, and let cool.

Press the salt through a sieve or sifter to return it to a granulated consistency. Store in an airtight container in a cool, dry place.

note

Don't use fancy salts like Himalayan pink or Maldon, as the tincture liquid will affect the shape and texture of the salt grains.

CBD FLAVORED BUTTERS

One thing I quickly discovered when cooking with hemp is that the pungent vegetal smell and flavor is very distinct. Making delicious things that meld well with its natural flavor is one of the challenges of cooking with cannabis, as it is strong and requires balancing. Think spicy, sweet, and citrus when making your own flavor combinations. I've also found that adding the CBD butter toward the end of cooking, or serving it as a condiment, works great. I like a 1:1 ratio of plain butter to infused, but feel free to experiment not only with the ratio, but with different flavors.

SPICY-SWEET CBD BUTTER

This one is great with chicken, pork, vegetables, and Asian noodles.

MAKES ABOUT 1 CUP

- 1 stick (½ cup) unsalted butter, softened
- 6 to 8 tablespoons CBD Butter (page 7)
- 1 tablespoon gochujang or sriracha hot sauce
- 1 teaspoon lime zest, or to taste
- 1 teaspoon honey or agave nectar, or to taste
- Pinch ground coriander
- Salt, to taste

In a small bowl, mix all ingredients until combined. Store in a glass container in the fridge.

SAGE CBD BUTTER

I like to serve this butter with poultry, on mashed potatoes, in gravy, or spread on French bread. It's especially good for relaxation on Thanksgiving!

MAKES ABOUT 1 CUP

- 1 stick (½ cup) unsalted butter, softened
- 6 to 8 tablespoons CBD Butter (page 7)
- 1 teaspoon dried or 1 tablespoon minced fresh sage
- ¼ teaspoon dried oregano
- ¼ teaspoon fennel seed, crushed (optional)
- ¼ teaspoon celery seed (optional)
- Dash red pepper flakes, or to taste

In a small bowl, mix all ingredients until combined. Store in a glass container in the fridge.

AUTUMN SPICE CBD BUTTER

Baked squash, French toast, baked apples, and roast pork would benefit from the warming spice of this butter. Try crushed fennel seed, freshly grated nutmeg, or ground coriander for different flavor profiles.

MAKES ABOUT 1 CUP

1	stick (½ cup) unsalted butter, softened
6 to 8	tablespoons CBD Butter (page 7)
1	tablespoon minced orange zest
1	tablespoon ground cinnamon
1	teaspoon ground cardamom
1	teaspoon ground ginger
	Large pinch salt
1	tablespoon honey or agave nectar

In a small bowl, mix all ingredients until combined. Store in a glass container in the fridge.

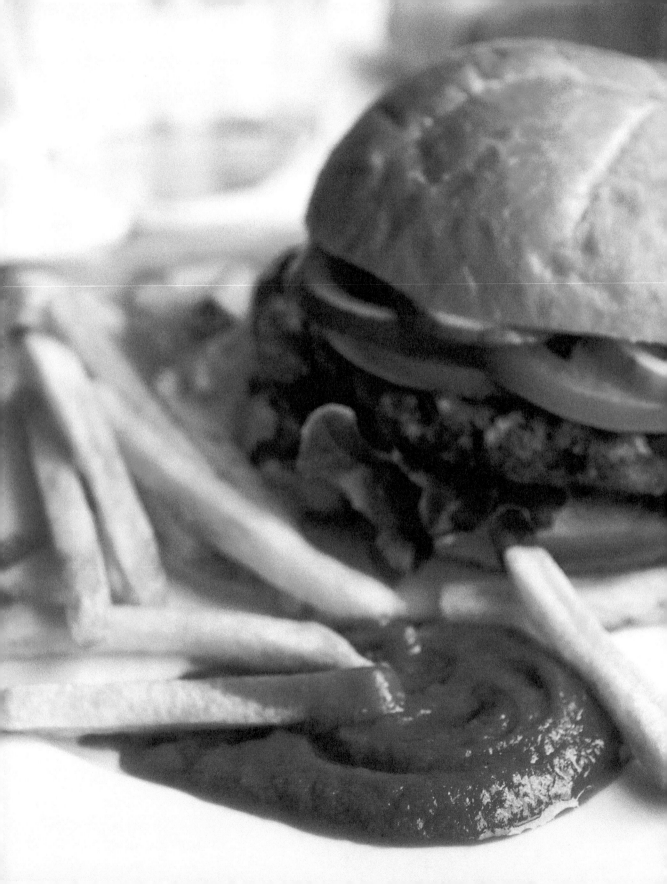

CBD KETCHUP

Ketchup is such a ubiquitous condiment—why not enjoy it medicated? The optional chipotle powder gives the sauce more of a smoky, BBQ flavor, and the anchovies will add complexity and umami.

½ cup water

1 small can (6 ounces) tomato paste

2 tablespoons apple cider vinegar

1 tablespoon CBD Olive Oil or Coconut Oil (page 7)

1 tablespoon brown sugar (light or dark)

1 teaspoon salt

1 teaspoon garlic powder

1 teaspoon onion powder

½ teaspoon anchovy paste (optional)

½ teaspoon chipotle powder (optional)

In a medium saucepan, whisk all of the ingredients to combine. Bring to a low boil over medium-high heat. As soon as it comes to the low boil, immediately turn it down to the lowest simmer. Cover the pan and cook, 30 to 60 minutes, or until thickened. (Remember, keep the heat very low so as not to cook off the CBD.) Remove from the heat and cool completely in the pan.

Store in a glass container in the fridge for up to 6 months.

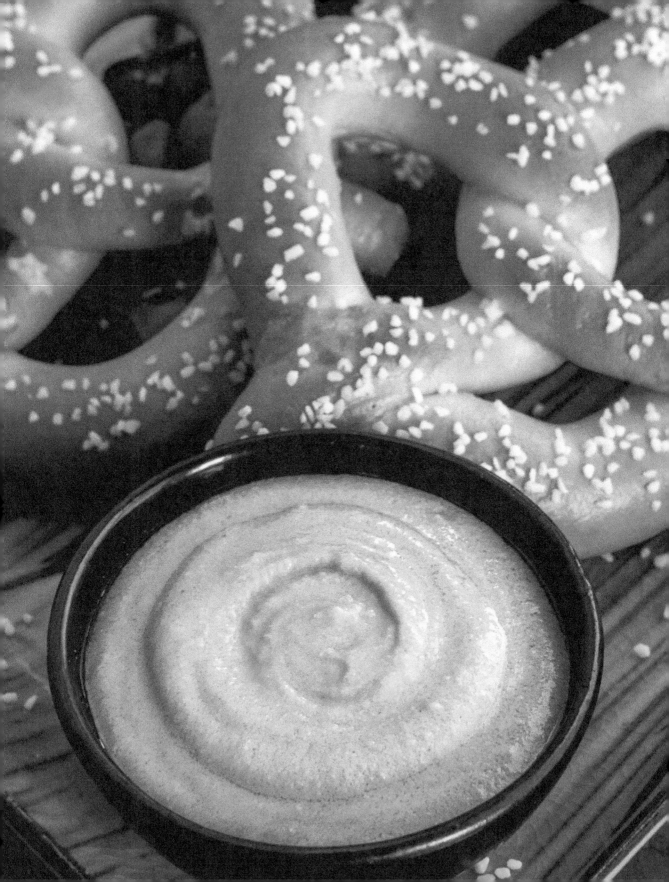

CBD SPICY MUSTARD

This mustard will add spice and fun to anything you use it on. Your hamburgers—and your guests—will thank you!

¼ cup water

4 tablespoons dry mustard (I use Colman's)

3 tablespoons white vinegar

1 tablespoon CBD Olive Oil (page 7)

½ teaspoon salt

¼ teaspoon garlic powder

¼ teaspoon ground turmeric

In a small saucepan, whisk all the ingredients to combine. Simmer over medium heat until the mixture thickens, about 5 minutes. Remove from the heat and cool completely in the pan.

Store in a glass container in the fridge for up to 6 months.

CBD MAYONNAISE

Once you make this a couple of times, you'll find that making mayo is easy and fun! I love that with little changes, you can have tons of variations. Use only olive oil for heartier food, a mix of oils for more complex flavors, or replace the vinegar with lemon juice. Add finely chopped herbs for a fresh taste, try curry powder and garam masala for a delicious curried chicken salad, or mix in diced pickles and some capers for a tasty tartar sauce.

MAKES 2 CUPS

- 2 egg yolks, room temperature (see Note)
- 1 tablespoon fresh lemon juice
- 2 teaspoons white vinegar
- 1 teaspoon Dijon mustard or CBD Spicy Mustard (page 19)
- 2 teaspoons salt, or to taste
- 1 cup canola or grapeseed oil
- ½ cup CBD Olive Oil (page 7)

In a food processor or blender, combine the yolks, lemon juice, vinegar, mustard, and salt. Process until blended and yellow, about 1 minute. With the motor running, very slowly add the oil in a thin stream until fully combined and the mayo is thick and smooth.

Store in a glass container in the fridge, and use within 2 days.

note
When making mayonnaise, always bring ingredients to room temperature, as warmer oil and eggs emulsify better.

CBD MAPLE SYRUP

This is another lovely way to get CBD into your food while keeping the cannabis flavor subtle. You can adjust it according to your taste and it's always delicious. Don't use artificial pancake syrup: You deserve the good stuff!

MAKES 1 CUP

1 cup dark or Grade B pure maple syrup

1 tablespoon to ½ cup CBD Glycerin Tincture (page 10)

1 tablespoon unsalted butter (extra points for CBD Butter, page 7)

Combine all the ingredients in a small saucepan. Warm gently over low heat, stirring occasionally, until all of the ingredients are incorporated.

Store in a glass container in the fridge for up to 6 months.

CBD HONEY

Honey—that wonderful gift from the bees—can easily carry your CBD without affecting the flavor. It's wonderful on biscuits, waffles, in tea . . . anywhere honey is your friend. Try it this way first, then add more tincture to taste.

MAKES 1 CUP

1 cup honey

2 tablespoons CBD Glycerin Tincture (page 10)

Seeds scraped from 1 vanilla bean, or ⅛ teaspoon vanilla extract (optional)

Place all the ingredients in a small jar with a lid. Close the lid. Place the jar in a saucepan, and add warm water till it comes halfway up the side of the jar. Warm over low heat for 5 minutes— don't let it boil. Remove the jar, stir the honey to blend, and cool completely. Store in the jar in a cool, dark place.

CBD NUT BUTTER

I, for one, am addicted to nut butters—I'll put them in a smoothie, on toast, wherever. The addition of infused coconut oil makes these spreads even better. Use peanut, cashew, or almond—or go crazy and mix them up!

MAKES 2 CUPS

2 cups roasted unsalted nuts

3 tablespoons CBD Coconut Oil (page 7)

½ teaspoon salt, or to taste

1 teaspoon brown sugar (light or dark, optional)

Place the nuts in a blender or food processor, and grind until they're almost smooth, scraping down the sides of the blender or processor when necessary. (This can take a while, so be patient!) When it's almost smooth, add the oil, salt, and sugar if using and blend until smooth.

Store in a glass container in the fridge.

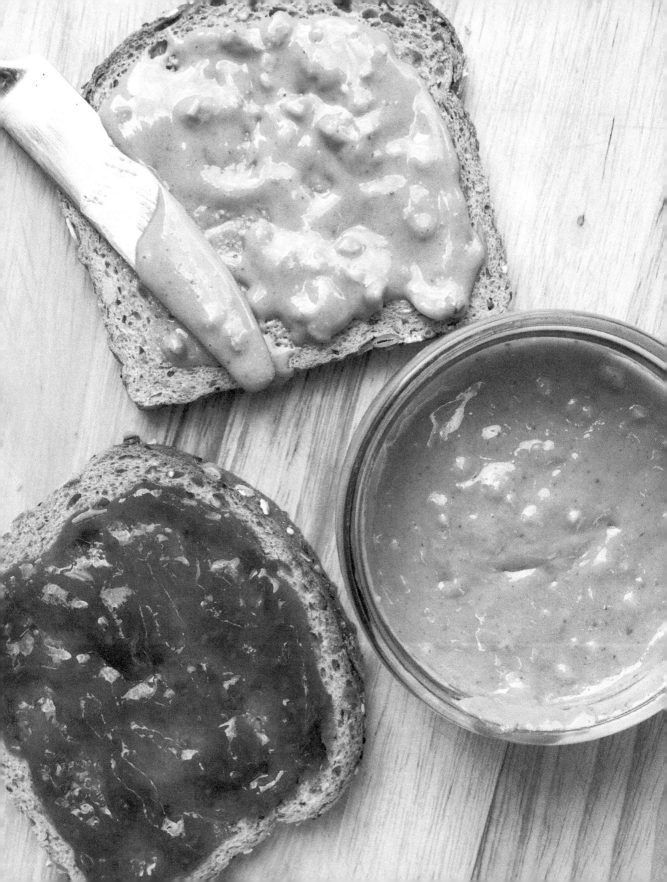

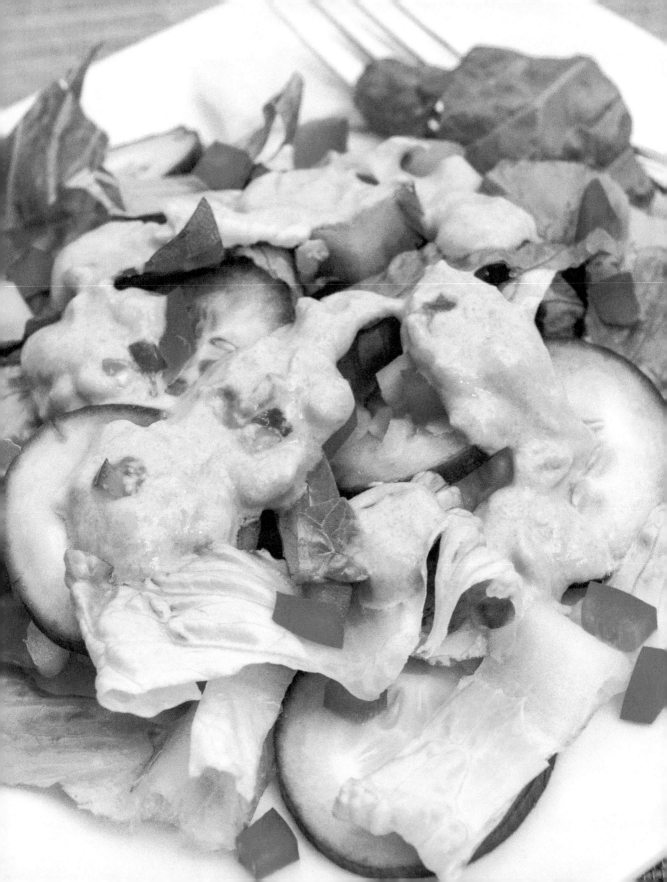

CBD SPECIAL SAUCE

This is a lovely salad dressing (like Thousand Island) or a great accompaniment to burgers. You'll love its tangy taste!

½ cup whole milk Greek yogurt

½ cup mayonnaise

½ cup ketchup

2 tablespoons CBD Olive Oil (page 7)

⅓ cup finely chopped pickles

Salt and freshly ground black pepper, to taste

Garlic powder, to taste

Pickle juice, to taste

Add all of the ingredients except the pickle juice to a quart-size jar. Close the lid and shake well until combined. Taste the dressing, adjust the seasoning, and stir in a tablespoon or two of pickle juice, until the dressing is the desired consistency.

Store in a glass container in the fridge for up to a month.

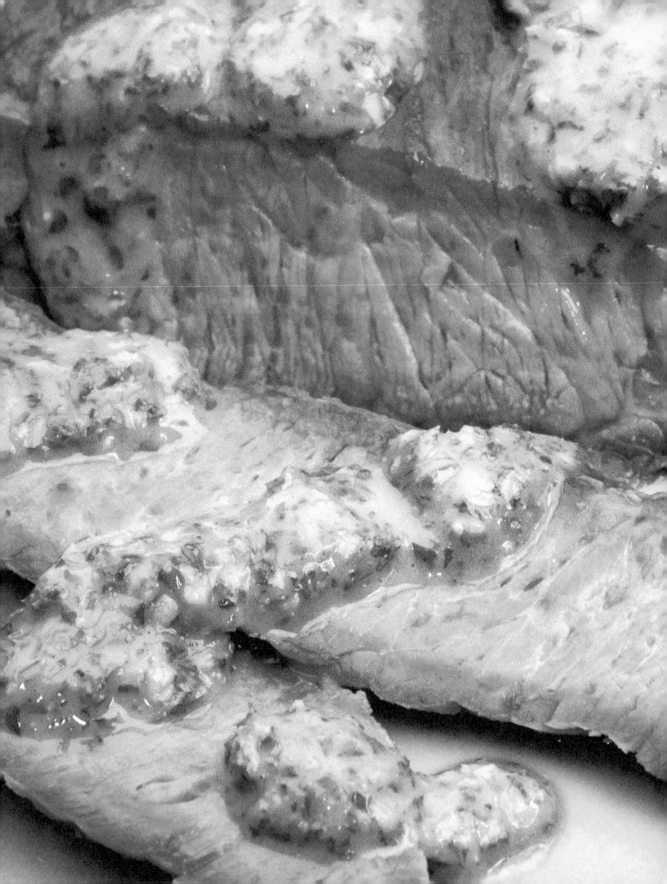

CBD CHIMICHURRI

This is a great addition to your grilling repertoire, as it livens up anything you cook over an open flame. I even use it as a topping for my Greenest Minestrone (page 73). It's a vacation to Argentina for your mouth!

MAKES ABOUT 1 CUP

1 cup packed fresh parsley leaves

3 large garlic cloves, chopped

2 tablespoons fresh or 1 tablespoon dried oregano

½ cup CBD Olive Oil (page 7) (or half CBD and half plain)

2 tablespoons red wine vinegar

½ teaspoon red pepper flakes, or to taste

Salt and freshly ground black pepper

In a food processor, pulse the parsley, garlic, and oregano together or chop finely by hand. Scrape into a small bowl. Stir in the rest of the ingredients to combine, adjust the seasoning with salt and pepper to taste, and serve.

Store in an airtight container in the fridge and use within 1 week.

CBD GRAVY

So many foods benefit from the addition of gravy. Chicken, meatloaf, biscuits, toasted bread—I mean, what *isn't* better with gravy? With this CBD version, you'll be happy and relaxed after enjoying it with your dinner. Swap in the Sage CBD Butter (page 14), which goes especially well with poultry.

2 tablespoons unsalted butter

1 small onion, minced

3 tablespoons all-purpose flour

2 tablespoons pan drippings or chicken or beef bouillon

1½ to 2 cups richly flavored stock, or 1½ cups stock and ½ cup wine

Salt and freshly ground black pepper

1 tablespoon CBD Butter (page 7)

In a large skillet over medium heat, melt the unsalted butter. Add the onion and cook until translucent, 7 to 9 minutes. Sprinkle the flour over the onion and butter and whisk for a few minutes until golden. Slowly add the drippings and stock, whisking constantly to prevent lumps. Cook for about 5 minutes or until the gravy begins to thicken. (If you use wine, cook a bit longer to evaporate the alcohol.) Season with salt and pepper to taste, and continue to cook until gravy is the desired consistency. Whisk in the CBD butter. Serve immediately.

CBD VINAIGRETTE DRESSING

With this recipe, there's no reason to ever buy salad dressing again! A great rule of thumb to remember for vinaigrette: it's 3 to 1 ratio—in other words, 3 parts oil to 1 part acid.

MAKES 4 SERVINGS

1 small shallot, minced

2 teaspoons Dijon mustard

2 to 3 tablespoons fresh lemon juice or a combination of lemon juice and red wine vinegar

Salt and freshly ground black pepper

¼ cup CBD Olive Oil (page 7)

¼ cup olive oil

Place the shallot, mustard, lemon juice, and salt and pepper to taste in a jar and shake vigorously to combine. Slowly add in the oils, whisking or shaking until combined.

Store in a glass container in the fridge.

STARTERS

SALSA FRESCA

A fresh, homemade salsa can really improve a meal, especially when it's Taco Tuesday. What's more, salsa does not have to be complicated to be delicious. This salsa fresca is best when made in season, with perfectly ripe tomatoes. Serve with chips, tacos, scrambled eggs—or really anything you like.

SERVES 4

3 large fresh tomatoes, diced

1 small red onion, finely diced

1 small jalapeño pepper, seeded and diced

Juice of one lime, or more to taste

Small bunch cilantro, chopped

1½ tablespoons CBD Olive Oil or Vegetable Oil (page 7)

Salt and freshly ground black pepper, to taste

Combine all ingredients in a bowl and stir well. Taste and adjust seasonings.

Store in a glass container in the fridge and allow the flavors to meld before serving.

GUACAMOLE

Guacamole . . . smooth, green, rich . . . what's not to love? This delicious version earns bonus points for helping you chill. This is a crowd pleaser, so get ready for your guac to disappear!

SERVES 6 TO 8

3 to 4   large ripe avocados

1   small jalapeño, seeded and finely diced (see Note)

½   small white onion, finely diced

1   tablespoon softened CBD Butter (page 7)

Juice and zest of 1 lime, or more as needed (see Note)

Salt and freshly ground black pepper

Halve, seed, and peel the avocados and put them in a bowl. Using a fork, smash the avocados until chunky. Add the remaining ingredients and mix well. Taste and adjust seasoning with salt and pepper to taste.

notes

Leave the seeds in the jalapeño if you like it hotter.

Sprinkle a little extra lime juice on top if it's going to sit out—this will help prevent browning.

HUMMUS

Making your own hummus is so easy and so much better than store-bought. Everyone loves hummus, and with CBD, well . . . it's the best! Serve with veggies, crackers, or wedges of pita bread.

SERVES 8

½ to ¾ cup CBD Vegetable Oil (page 7)

One 15.5-ounce can garbanzo beans (chickpeas), drained and rinsed

¾ cup tahini (sesame paste)

3 to 4 tablespoons fresh lemon juice

2 to 3 cloves garlic, chopped

2 teaspoons cumin

Salt and freshly ground black pepper, to taste

Red pepper flakes, to taste

Chopped parsley or roasted red pepper strips, for garnish

Into the bowl of a food processor, place ½ cup of the CBD oil and remaining ingredients except the garnishes. Process at least 2 minutes and up to 6 minutes, until the desired consistency, adding more CBD oil to thin if needed. Remove the hummus to a bowl, garnish with parsley or roasted pepper, and serve.

WHITE BEAN DIP

This creamy, hearty dip is a perfect last-minute appetizer since it's made with ingredients you usually have on hand. Don't have cannellini beans? Navy and Great Northern beans work well too. Serve with toasted bread, crackers, or veggies for dipping.

MAKES ABOUT 2 CUPS

One 15.5-ounce can cannellini beans, drained and rinsed see Headnote)

1 to 3 cloves garlic, minced

2 tablespoons CBD Olive Oil (page 7)

Salt, to taste

Red pepper flakes, to taste

Juice and zest of one large lemon, some zest reserved

½ teaspoon finely minced fresh rosemary, some reserved

In a blender or a food processor, process the beans a little—they should still be chunky. Add remaining ingredients except the reserved zest and rosemary, and process to combine. The consistency should be smooth with a few chunks. Remove to a bowl and garnish with the reserved rosemary and zest. Serve with your favorite dippers.

DEVILED EGGS

This is a classic that is only improved with the addition of calming, healthful CBD. Try topping the eggs with different garnishes for a colorful, festive platter. Like them spicy? Sprinkle with cayenne instead of paprika. Swapping in CBD Mayonnaise (page 20) is another good opportunity to add more CBD.

MAKES 12 DEVILED EGGS

6 large eggs

2 teaspoons CBD Olive Oil (page 7)

¼ cup mayonnaise

1 tablespoon full-fat Greek yogurt

1 tablespoon Dijon mustard or CBD Spicy Mustard (page 19)

Salt and freshly ground black pepper

Capers, paprika, smoked chili powder, or chopped chives, for garnish

Place the eggs in a medium saucepan with enough cold water to cover. Bring just to a rolling boil over high heat, remove from the heat, and cover. Let stand for 20 minutes, then plunge the eggs into a bowl full of ice—*voilà*, perfect hardboiled eggs. Peel eggs and cut them in half carefully. Set the whites aside.

Place the yolks in a medium bowl. Add the remaining ingredients except the garnishes and mash and mix the filling until smooth. Taste and adjust seasoning with salt and pepper to taste. (Play around with this—if it's too dry and crumbly, add more mayo or yogurt for more creaminess.) Using a teaspoon, fill the egg halves with the yolk mixture. Garnish to taste.

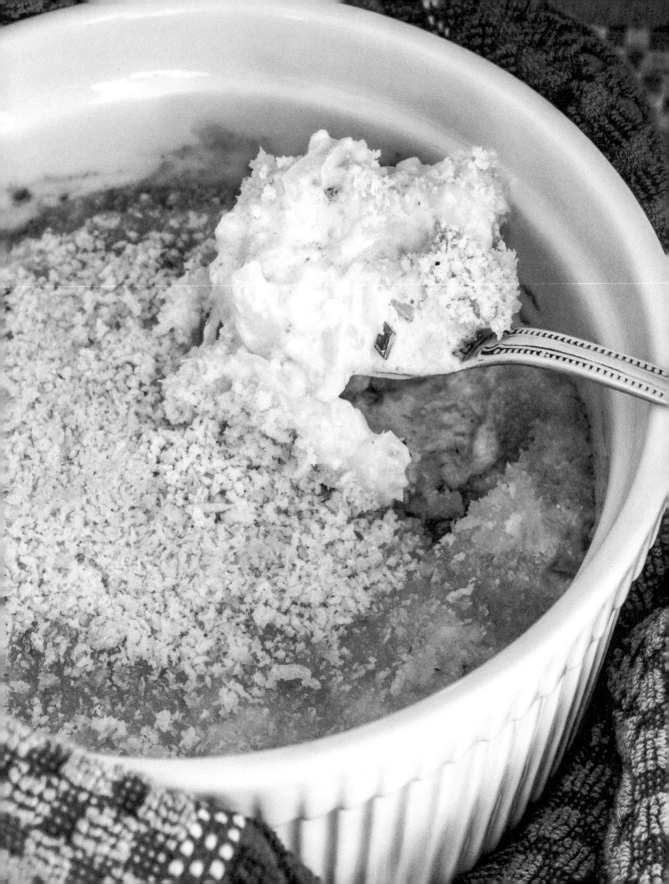

BAKED ARTICHOKE DIP

This is a classic and well worth having in your appetizer arsenal. Everyone enjoys it, and you can tell yourself you're basically eating vegetables. . . .

1 cup finely grated Parmesan

¾ cup mayonnaise

½ cup finely chopped sweet onion

3 tablespoons CBD Butter (page 7), softened

One 14-ounce can artichoke hearts, well drained

1 tablespoon fresh lemon juice

Salt and freshly ground black pepper

½ cup plain dry breadcrumbs or panko

Olive oil

Preheat the oven to 400°F. In a medium bowl, stir together the Parmesan, mayonnaise, onions, and butter. Place the artichoke hearts in a food processor and process until finely chopped. Add the artichokes, lemon juice, and salt and pepper to taste to the cheese mixture. Stir to combine, then spread into a small baking dish, sprinkle with the breadcrumbs, and lightly drizzle with olive oil. Bake until the top is golden, about 20 minutes, and serve warm with crackers or crostini.

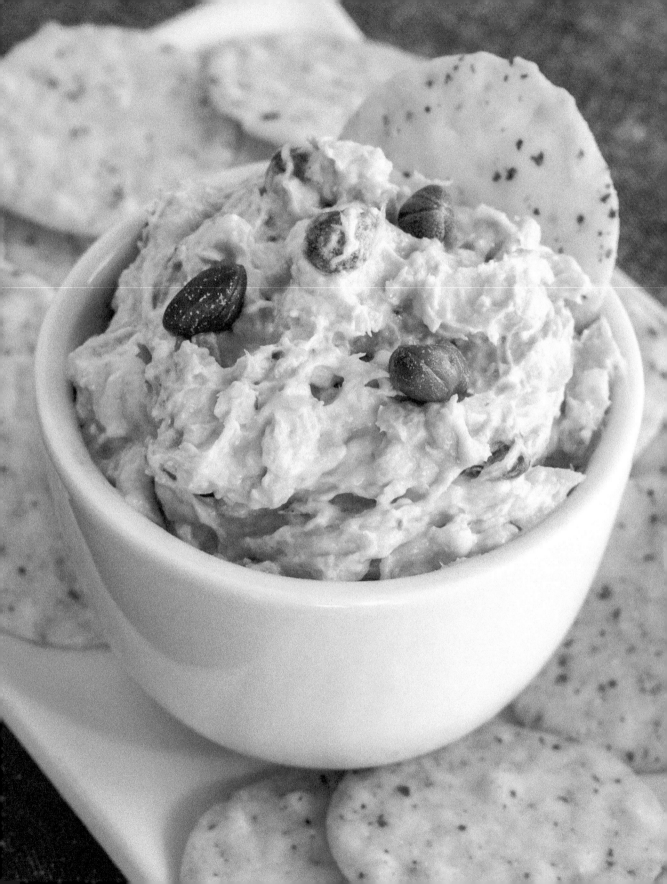

SALMON SPREAD

Normally I don't use canned salmon, but in this case it's really good. Just be sure to get the canned wild red (sockeye) salmon. Pink or farmed salmon won't have the same flavor. This tasty dip has served us well at many a get-together. It's delightful with champagne.

MAKES 3 CUPS

Two 6-ounce cans skinless boneless red (sockeye) salmon

Two 8-ounce packages cream cheese, softened

½ cup mayonnaise

3 tablespoons CBD Butter (page 7), softened

¼ red onion, minced

Zest of 1 lemon

Salt and freshly ground black pepper, to taste

2 tablespoons drained small capers (optional)

Combine all the ingredients in a bowl, mix well, and chill until about an hour before you want to serve. Bring it to room temperature and serve with raw vegetables, crackers, or pita chips.

SPICY NUTS

Talk about a great party starter! These spicy nuts are deliciously irresistible, so you and your guests may be tempted to eat too many and ruin your dinners.

2 cups unsalted almonds or mixed nuts

1 tablespoon brown sugar (light or dark)

1 teaspoon ground cumin

1 teaspoon smoked paprika

½ teaspoon garlic powder

½ teaspoon salt

1 tablespoon CBD Olive Oil (page 7)

1 tablespoon CBD Alcohol Tincture (page 10)

In a dry skillet, toast the nuts over medium heat until they show some color, 3 to 4 minutes. Set them aside in a serving bowl. In a small bowl, mix the brown sugar, cumin, paprika, garlic, and salt. In the same skillet over medium-low heat, gently warm the oil, add the spice mixture, and cook, stirring, for less than a minute. (Too much heat will affect the CBD in the oil and tincture, so be careful here.) Remove the pan from the heat and add the toasted nuts and the tincture, stirring to coat evenly.

Serve warm or at room temperature. Store in an airtight container.

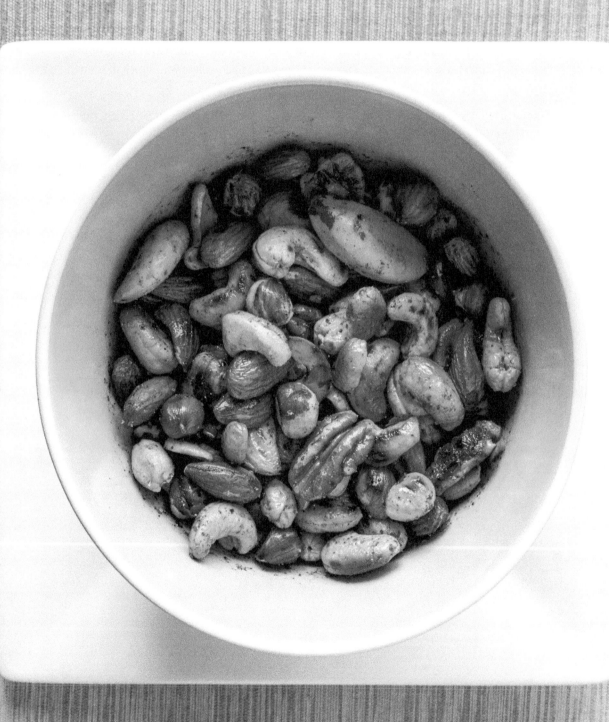

GARLIC BREAD

Who doesn't love warm, buttery garlic bread with soup, stew, chili, pasta dishes, or just topped with cheese and broiled? This delightful loaf will complete your lunch or dinner.

MAKES 1 LOAF

1	loaf best-quality French, country, or sourdough bread
3 or 4	garlic cloves, minced or pressed
½	cup CBD Butter (page 7) or 4 tablespoons CBD butter plus 4 tablespoons butter, softened
	Sea salt, or any fancy salt you like

Preheat the oven to 400°F. Slice the bread diagonally into 10 to 12 slices, without cutting through the loaf completely. Combine the garlic and butter, stirring until incorporated. Spread each side of the slices with the garlic butter and squish the loaf back together. Sprinkle the top with salt to taste, wrap in foil, and bake 15 to 20 minutes or until the loaf is crisp and brown on top and your house smells great. Serve hot.

CHERRY TOMATOES *with* BLUE CHEESE

These little bites are super easy to make, elegant, and actually pretty good for you. For a delicious vegetarian version, swap the bacon for toasted walnuts.

MAKES 2 DOZEN

24 cherry tomatoes, washed and stemmed

½ cup crumbled blue cheese

1 tablespoon CBD Butter (page 7)

4 slices crisp bacon, crumbled, or 24 toasted walnut halves

Chopped fresh chives or sliced green onion tops, for garnish

Carefully carve out a cavity inside of each tomato with a paring knife or melon baller and gently squeeze out some of the seeds. In a small bowl, mix the blue cheese and butter until incorporated. Press about a teaspoon of the cheese mixture into the cavity of each tomato, then top with bacon or a walnut. Arrange cheese side up on a serving platter, garnish with chives or green onions, and serve.

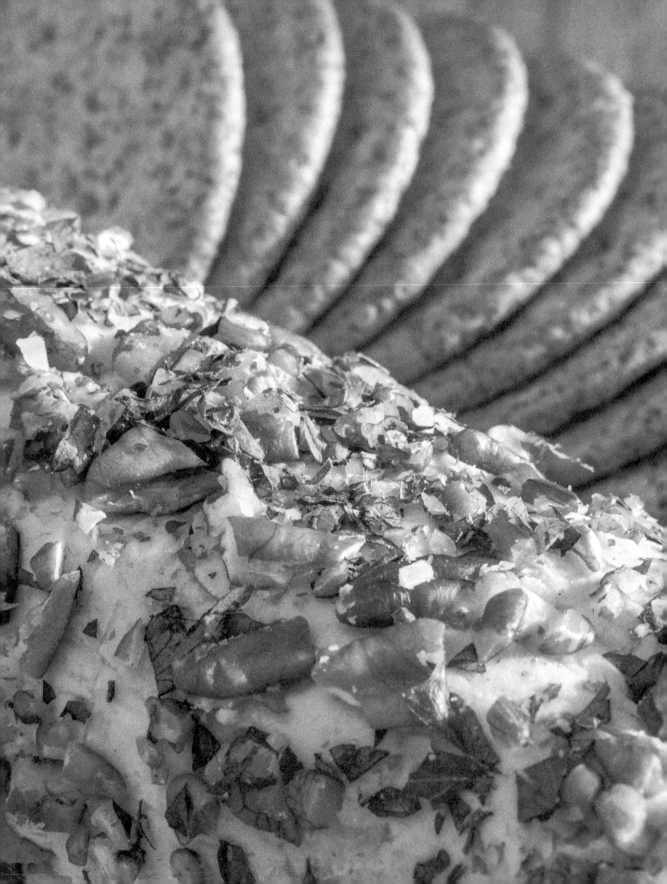

CLASSIC CHEESE LOGS

Sometimes a delicious old-school cheese log (or ball) is just the thing. This recipe, when made with CBD butter, guarantees a very relaxed dinner party. Plus it freezes well, so you can have it on hand whenever you need a cheese fix (see Note).

MAKES 2 LOGS; SERVES 12

Two 8-ounce packages of cream cheese, softened

1 tablespoon Worcestershire sauce

1 clove garlic, finely minced

Dash red pepper flakes, or to taste

4 cups grated sharp cheddar

6 to 8 tablespoons CBD Butter (page 7)

1 teaspoon salt

½ cup toasted pecans, finely chopped

¼ cup finely minced parsley

In a food processor, combine the cream cheese, Worcestershire, garlic, and red pepper flakes to taste and process until well blended. Add the cheese and butter and pulse until all the cheese is incorporated but bits are still visible. Form the mixture into 2 logs about 6 inches long (or two balls), wrap tightly in plastic wrap, and chill until firm. While the logs are chilling, mix the pecans and parsley together, and when the logs are firm, roll them in the nut/parsley mix.

note

Want to make these ahead? Before rolling in the nut mixture, wrap the logs well in plastic wrap and chill for at least an hour or until you need them. They also will keep in the freezer, wrapped in two layers of freezer wrap, for about a month. When the cheese log urge strikes, defrost in the fridge until slightly soft (a couple of hours), and roll in the nut mixture before serving.

BURNT STONE FRUIT
with CHEESE

This is my take on a version of a recipe I originally saw in *Bon Appétit*. You'll be amazed at how good burnt fruit can be. This is lovely as an appetizer or even a dessert—your choice!

SERVES 4 TO 6

8 ounces soft goat cheese

2 teaspoons CBD Glycerin Tincture (page 10)

2 tablespoons unsalted butter

1 tablespoon CBD Butter (page 7)

6 plums, peaches, nectarines, or other stone fruit, halved and pitted

Salt and freshly ground black pepper

CBD Olive Oil (page 7)

In a small bowl, mix the goat cheese and tincture until combined. Set aside. Melt the butters in a skillet over medium heat and cook until the foam subsides. Add the fruit, cut side down. Cook for at least 5 minutes, ensuring the cut sides get charred. Place the hot fruit cut side up on a serving platter and let cool a little. Crumble the goat cheese mixture over the fruit, sprinkle with salt and pepper to taste, and drizzle with CBD oil. Serve immediately.

STUFFED 'SHROOMS
with BÉCHAMEL

I adapted this recipe from the incredible Marcella Hazan, and it's wonderful. Savory, elegant, and bite-sized, these mushrooms are perfect party finger food. Leave the prosciutto or ham out for a vegetarian version.

SERVES 6

BÉCHAMEL SAUCE

- 1½ tablespoons butter
- 1½ tablespoons all-purpose flour
- 1 teaspoon salt
- 1 cup milk, warmed

STUFFED 'SHROOMS

- 12 large mushrooms, wiped clean, stems removed and finely chopped
- 1 tablespoon butter
- 2 tablespoons CBD Butter (page 7), divided
- 1 tablespoon minced onion or shallot
- 3 tablespoons chopped prosciutto or ham (optional)

   Salt and freshly ground black pepper
- 3 tablespoons freshly grated Parmesan

   Plain dry breadcrumbs

FOR THE BÉCHAMEL SAUCE: Melt the butter in a medium saucepan over medium-low heat. Slowly stir in the flour. Cook, stirring constantly to prevent lumps, until golden and nutty-smelling, 5 to 7 minutes. Add the salt and warm milk and whisk constantly to prevent lumps. When the mixture thickens, remove from the heat and set aside, stirring occasionally to prevent skin from forming.

FOR THE STUFFED 'SHROOMS: Preheat the oven to 500°F. Grease a large baking dish and add the mushroom caps, curved side down.

In a skillet over medium heat, melt 1 tablespoon of butter and 1 tablespoon of CBD butter. Add the onion and cook, stirring occasionally, until golden, about 5 minutes. Add the prosciutto, if using, and cook for about 1 minute. Add the chopped stems and salt and pepper to taste. Cook, stirring occasionally, for about 3 minutes or until the stems are soft and the prosciutto starts to brown. Tilt the skillet and discard most of the fat.

In a medium bowl, mix the mushroom mixture with the béchamel, add the Parmesan, and mix again. Sprinkle the mushroom caps lightly with salt, fill with the béchamel mixture, sprinkle with breadcrumbs, and dot with the remaining 1 tablespoon of CBD butter. Bake for 15 minutes; let cool a little, then serve warm.

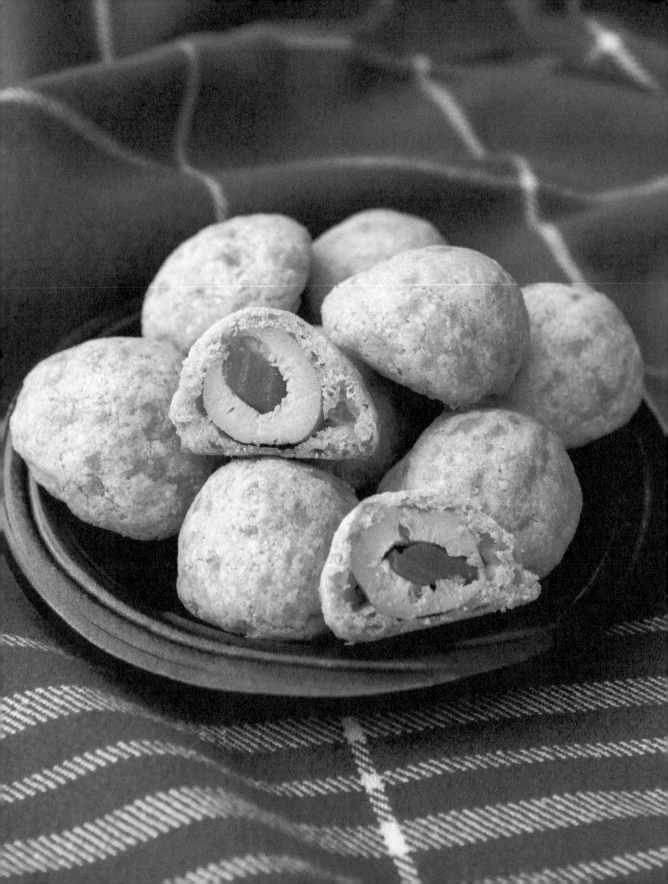

CHEESY OLIVE BITES

These are wonderful and have a great 1960s cocktail culture vibe. They're totally addictive with an adult beverage, so try not to eat them all!

MAKES 35 TO 40

2 cups finely grated cheddar

4 tablespoons CBD Butter (page 7), softened

1¼ cups all-purpose flour

Cayenne pepper

35 to 40 pimiento-stuffed olives, well-drained and patted dry (two 10-ounce jars)

Preheat the oven to 400°F. In a medium bowl, beat the cheese and butter together with a hand mixer until smooth. Add the flour and cayenne to taste, and mix until combined. Take about a teaspoon of dough, flatten it into a circle about ⅛ inch thick, and wrap it around each olive, forming a cute little coat. Roll between your palms to completely cover the olive. Place on an ungreased baking sheet and bake until firm and golden, about 15 minutes. Serve warm.

ASPARAGUS *and* PROSCIUTTO ROLLS

The combination of flavors in this recipe will make you and your friends very happy. They're salty, creamy, and wonderful.

SERVES 4 TO 6

1 pound fresh asparagus, ends trimmed

4 ounces cream cheese, softened

1 teaspoon CBD Olive Oil (page 7)

1 teaspoon CBD Butter (page 7), softened

4 ounces prosciutto, or good-quality sliced ham

Preheat the oven to 375°F. Line a baking sheet with parchment paper.

In a large pot of boiling water, blanch the asparagus for about 1 minute, then drain well. In a small bowl, mix together the cream cheese, oil, and butter. Lay out a slice of the prosciutto, spread it with 1 teaspoon of the cream cheese mixture, and then place an asparagus spear on one end and roll up. Repeat with the remaining ingredients. Place rolls on the baking sheet and bake for 10 to 12 minutes, or until the asparagus is still crisp and the prosciutto kind of crinkly. Remove to a serving platter and serve immediately.

ROASTED PEPPER ROLL-UPS

This is a lovely pepper preparation from Sicily. To make this vegan, substitute 2 tablespoons finely diced, sautéed mushrooms for the anchovies.

SERVES 4

3   medium red and yellow bell peppers

3   tablespoons olive oil

⅓   cup plain dry breadcrumbs

2   tablespoons toasted pine nuts

2   tablespoons raisins, soaked in warm water for 15 minutes and drained (see Note)

2   anchovies, finely chopped

1½   tablespoons capers, drained and chopped

1   tablespoon minced parsley

   Salt and freshly ground black pepper

¼   cup CBD Olive Oil (page 7)

Preheat the broiler. Coat the peppers with the oil and broil, turning often until the skin is blackened all over. Remove and let cool, then rub the peppers to remove the charred skins—they should peel right off. Cut each pepper into quarters, remove the stem and seeds, and set aside.

Preheat the oven to 425°F. In a small bowl, combine the breadcrumbs, pine nuts, raisins, anchovies, capers, parsley, and salt and pepper to taste. Taste and adjust the seasoning, and stir in the oil. Lay out the sliced peppers insides-up. Divide the breadcrumb mixture among them, placing it at the wide end of each slice. Roll up each slice and secure with a toothpick. Place on a baking sheet and bake for 15 minutes or until the breadcrumbs look browned and crispy. Serve hot or at room temperature.

note

For more CBD, add 1 tablespoon CBD Alcohol Tincture (page 10) to the raisin soaking water, soak up to 30 minutes, and drain.

SAUSAGES *with* SWEET-SOUR FIGS

Every time I make these, I thank the wonderful cookbook author Penelope Casas because they're dee-licious! You do need to marinate the figs a day ahead, but they're definitely worth the wait. Use large, firm link sausages like sweet Italian or Merguez (from North Africa). These can be made ahead and reheated as needed (see Note).

SERVES 8

FIGS

- 1 cup granulated sugar
- 1 cup red wine vinegar
- 1 tablespoon CBD Alcohol Tincture (page 10)
- 1 stick cinnamon
- 4 cloves
- 1 slice lemon
- 1 pound fresh figs (25 to 30)

SAUSAGES

- 1 tablespoon CBD Olive Oil (page 7)
- 4 tablespoons white wine, divided
- 1½ pounds sausage links
- 2 teaspoons tomato paste

  Salt and freshly ground black pepper

FOR THE FIGS: In a saucepan, combine the all the ingredients except the figs. Over medium-high heat, bring the mixture just to a boil, then turn the heat to low and simmer for 5 minutes, or until the liquid has thickened slightly. Add the figs and simmer for 20 more minutes. Cool and let marinate at least 4 hours or overnight in the fridge.

FOR THE SAUSAGES: In a skillet over medium heat, heat the oil and 2 tablespoons of the wine. Reduce the heat to medium-low, add the sausages, and cook until the wine evaporates and the sausages are cooked through. Remove the sausages to a warm platter and pour off most of the fat from the pan. Deglaze the pan with 4 tablespoons water and the remaining 2 tablespoons of wine. Add the tomato paste and salt and pepper to taste, stir, and simmer for 2 to 3 minutes. Drain the figs and add them and the sausages to the pan. Cover and cook briefly until the figs are heated through.

To serve, cut each sausage into 3 or 4 pieces. Slice the figs in half or quarters, depending on their size. Spear a piece of fig and sausage on each toothpick, place on a serving platter with the sauce, and serve.

note

The bites can also be assembled in advance and reheated, covered, at 300°F for 30 minutes or until warmed through.

EGG FRITTERS (PISCI D'OVU)

These are magical puffs of goodness, and make for a fabulous appetizer. This is an Italian classic adapted from the queen of Italian cooking, Marcella Hazan.

SERVES 6

1 tablespoon CBD Sage Butter (page 14)

1 tablespoon unsalted butter

4 eggs

2 tablespoons freshly grated Parmesan

½ teaspoon garlic, minced

½ cup plain dry breadcrumbs

Salt and freshly ground black pepper

Vegetable oil, for frying

In a small bowl, mix the CBD butter with the unsalted butter and set aside. Break the eggs into a medium bowl and beat them lightly. Add the Parmesan, garlic, breadcrumbs, and salt and pepper to taste and mix until combined.

Add enough oil to a deep skillet to make a depth of 1 inch, and heat it over medium-high heat. When the oil is hot (a drop of batter will stiffen and float), add the batter a teaspoonful at a time, being careful not to crowd the pan. When the fritters puff up and are golden on one side, turn them and cook until golden. Transfer to a paper towel or a cooling rack to drain. Serve immediately with the butter mixture on the side.

OLIVE SHORTBREAD

These are buttery and delicious; both savory and sweet!. You can substitute Kalamata or green olives for the cured olives; just make sure to thoroughly dry them before mixing them into the dough.

1 cup CBD Butter (page 7), softened

2 tablespoons packed light brown sugar

2¼ cups all-purpose flour

1 teaspoon salt

1 cup oil-cured olives, thoroughly dried, pitted, and chopped

Preheat the oven to 350°F. Grease a 9-inch square baking pan. In the bowl of a stand mixer, beat the butter and sugar until creamy, about 2 minutes. Reduce the speed to low, add the flour and salt, and beat just to combine. Fold in the olives and then smooth the dough into the pan, pressing it in firmly. Prick all over with a fork to prevent puffing. Bake until golden brown and pulling away from the edges, about 30 minutes. Cool completely in the pan, then cut into 1½–inch squares.

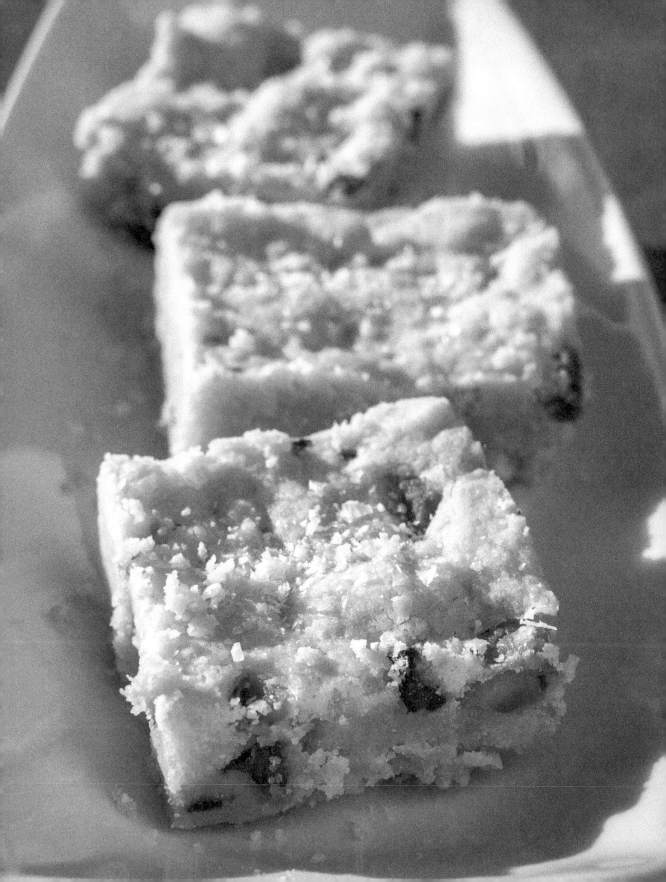

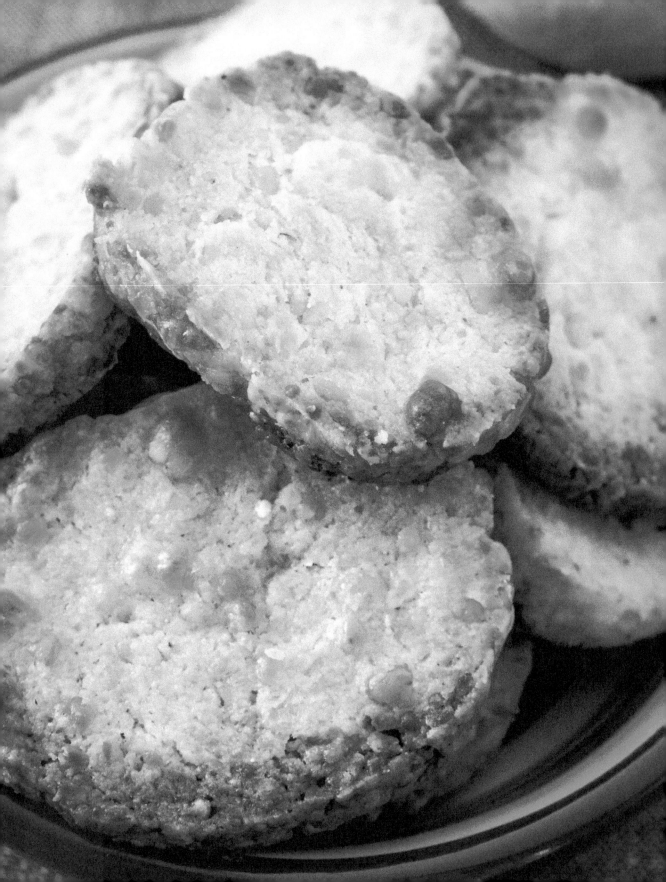

LEMON COCKTAIL CRACKERS

These crackers are great with cheeses and cured meats, plus you can make them ahead—freeze the dough log and bake off the crackers as needed (see Note). These are so good, it's worth making your own crackers!

MAKES ABOUT 3½ DOZEN

1½ cups finely grated Parmesan

¾ cup all-purpose flour

1 teaspoon finely grated lemon zest

1 teaspoon freshly ground black pepper

4 tablespoons CBD Butter (page 7), cold and cut into ½-inch pieces

1½ tablespoons water

1 teaspoon lemon juice

2 teaspoons salt

In a large bowl, whisk together the Parmesan, flour, lemon zest, and pepper. Add the butter and cut it in, until the mixture is crumbly with some larger pea-sized pieces. Make a well in the center and add the remaining ingredients. Stir with a fork until it begins to come together, then briefly knead until just combined into a dough. On a sheet of parchment paper, shape the dough into a log about 2 inches in diameter. Chill the dough for at least an hour so it's firm enough to slice, or wrap well and refrigerate until needed (see Note). When you're ready to bake, preheat the oven to 375°F, slice these thin (about ⅛ inch), and bake for 10 minutes, or until golden around the edges.

note

If you want to make the dough ahead of time, wrap the log tightly in freezer wrap and refrigerate up to 5 days, or freeze for up to 3 months. Defrost in the fridge and prepare as above.

SALADS *and* SIDES

CHICKEN SALAD
with RADISHES

This unique chicken salad is probably tastier than what you're used to—the CBD mayo and crunch from pickles and radishes makes it sing! Serve over mixed greens, or use it to make a decadent, gooey chicken melt sandwich.

SERVES 4

2 cups chopped or shredded cooked chicken

1 bunch radishes, tops removed and sliced thin

½ cup cornichons or strong dill pickles, chopped

¾ cup CBD Mayonnaise (page 20)

2 tablespoons white vinegar

2 hard-boiled eggs, chopped or sliced

Salt and freshly ground black pepper

Finely chopped chives, fresh tarragon, or parsley, for garnish

In a large bowl, combine the chicken, radishes, and cornichons. In a small bowl, combine the mayo and vinegar, then add this to the chicken mixture and combine. Carefully fold in the eggs, season liberally with salt and pepper to taste, and garnish with the chopped herbs. Chill before serving to maximize crunch.

CAESAR SALAD

A good Caesar salad is a joy and one of my favorite things to eat. This is the classic, and the bright lemon flavor and umami-rich anchovies are a treat for your mouth.

4 to 6 anchovy fillets in oil, drained

2 egg yolks

2 tablespoons fresh lemon juice

1 large clove garlic, chopped

1 tablespoon Dijon mustard

1 tablespoon CBD Olive Oil (page 7)

½ cup olive oil

3 to 4 tablespoons freshly grated Parmesan, plus more for garnish

2 large heads Romaine lettuce, washed, dried, and roughly torn into pieces

CBD Croutons (recipe follows)

In a blender or food processor, process the anchovies, yolks, lemon juice, garlic, mustard, and CBD olive oil until combined. With the blender or food processor running, slowly add the plain olive oil in a thin stream. Blend until the dressing is thick and creamy, then add the cheese and pulse to combine. Remove to a glass container and set aside. Right before serving, place the Romaine in a large salad bowl, add about half of the dressing (or more to taste), and toss to coat. Top with the croutons and Parmesan.

CBD CROUTONS

I like to use hearty, dark bread for my croutons, but any good crusty baguette or country bread will work well. Day-old or slightly stale bread works best.

2 to 3   tablespoons CBD Olive Oil (page 7)

2 to 3   tablespoons olive oil

4 to 6   slices hearty, dark bread, cut into 1-inch cubes

2   teaspoons CBD Salt (page 13)

In a large skillet over medium-high heat, warm the olive oils. When the oil is hot and bubbling around the edges, add the bread cubes. Cook the bread in the oil, tossing occasionally, watching carefully to ensure all the cubes are toasted and golden and don't burn. This will take about 10 minutes. Remove to paper towels to drain and sprinkle with salt.

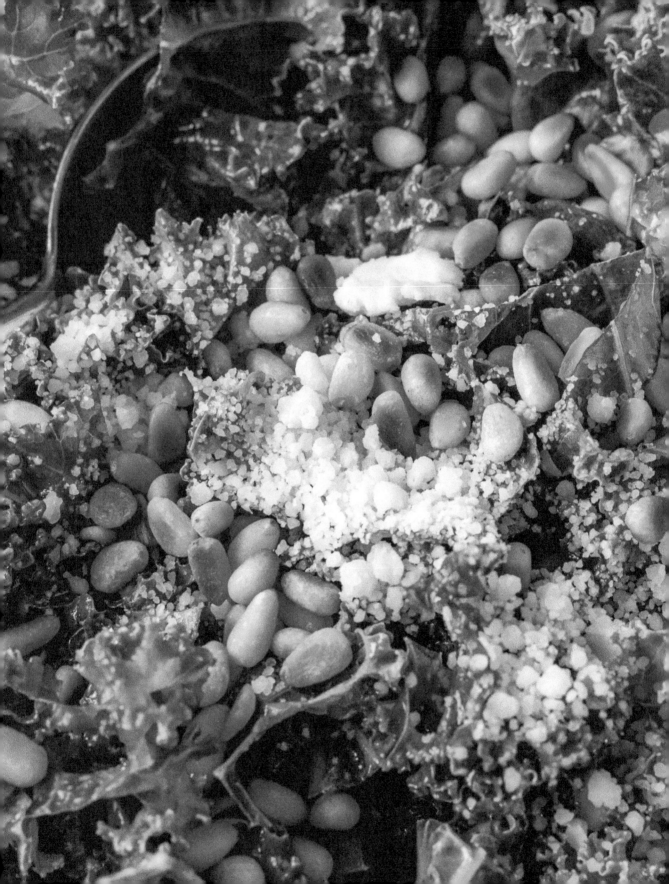

THE BEST KALE SALAD

Once you try this, you'll be one of those people who say, "I love kale!" This was inspired by a great salad I had at Tom Douglas's Serious Pie.

1 large bunch kale (dinosaur or lacinato)

2 tablespoons fresh lemon juice

1½ tablespoons CBD Olive Oil (page 7)

½ teaspoon Dijon mustard

Salt

1 Fresno or other hot pepper, seeded and finely diced

3 tablespoons toasted pine nuts

Freshly grated Pecorino Romano or Parmesan

Remove the kale stems and chop the leaves into bite-size pieces. In a large bowl, whisk together the lemon juice, oil, mustard, and a large pinch of salt. Add the kale to the bowl along with the hot pepper (add less if you prefer less heat) and toss to coat. Massage the dressing into the kale, then put it in the fridge to marinate for at least 30 minutes, taking it out about every 10 minutes to massage it as it's marinating. Don't skip this step—it really does make a difference. When it's chilled and ready to serve, divide the salad among 4 chilled plates and top with the pine nuts and cheese.

NETTER'S ASIAN CHICKEN SALAD

This tasty salad is easy, quick, healthy, and—oh yeah—seriously good! Serve it over fluffy brown rice for a hearty, filling meal.

SERVES 4 TO 6

2 cups water

½ cup soy sauce, plus more to taste

1 tablespoon red pepper flakes, or to taste

1½ pounds boneless, skinless chicken thighs, cut into small pieces

1 large head broccoli, cut into small pieces

1 seedless English cucumber, diced

2 to 3 scallions, thinly sliced (optional)

3 to 4 tablespoons peanut oil

1 tablespoon CBD Vegetable or Olive Oil (page 7)

1 to 2 tablespoons rice wine vinegar, or to taste

1 tablespoon toasted sesame oil

Toasted sesame seeds, for garnish

In a large saucepan over medium-low heat, combine the water, soy sauce, and pepper flakes and bring to a simmer. Add the chicken pieces, stir well, and keep at a simmer until cooked through, about 15 minutes. Add the broccoli and let it blanch for about 1 minute, until bright green and still crunchy. Remove from the heat into a large bowl, and let the chicken mixture cool for at least 20 minutes (or chill covered in the fridge until you're ready to serve). Add the remaining ingredients, combine well, and sprinkle with sesame seeds. Taste and season with more soy sauce, vinegar, or sesame to taste.

PERFECT PASTA SALAD

Forget everything you've ever read or thought about pasta salad—this one, adapted from the inimitable Marcella Hazan, does it perfectly. This is wonderful as a side dish or a light summer entrée with the addition of a protein.

SERVES 4 TO 6

1 pound thin spaghetti

¼ cup olive oil

1 dozen Kalamata olives, pitted

6 to 8 flat anchovy fillets

2 tablespoons drained small capers

Juice and zest of a large lemon, some zest reserved

2 tablespoons parsley, finely chopped

2 tablespoons CBD Olive Oil (page 7)

Salt and freshly ground black pepper

Cook the pasta until al dente. Drain, transfer to a bowl, and toss with the ¼ cup olive oil. Set aside to cool completely. Meanwhile, slice half the olives into thin strips and chop the rest into a fine pulp. In a large bowl, smash the anchovies into small pieces, then add the olives, capers, lemon juice and zest, and parsley. Add the pasta and toss until coated, and let it rest for about 30 minutes. Before serving, toss again with the CBD oil, taste and adjust seasoning with salt and pepper to taste, and sprinkle with reserved lemon zest.

GREEK-STYLE QUINOA

This salad can be changed up depending on who's coming over. Get creative and experiment with the vegetables, nuts, and cheeses that you add for alternative flavor combinations. Try some soaked and drained raisins, chopped cooked chicken, or even cubed firm tofu if you like. I find it's best enjoyed with a crisp white wine.

SERVES 8

1½ cups uncooked quinoa

2 cups stock or water

½ cup finely chopped red onion

1 cup pitted sliced Kalamata olives

½ cup crumbled feta cheese

½ cup toasted pine nuts

1 small zucchini, sliced into ribbons or finely diced

1 cup grape tomatoes, halved

3 tablespoons olive oil

1½ tablespoons CBD Olive Oil (page 7)

Juice of one lemon

Large handful fresh oregano, chopped

Salt and freshly ground black pepper, to taste

Cook the quinoa per package directions and cool. Place in a large mixing bowl and add the remaining ingredients. Toss to combine and serve.

SHAUN'S SUCCOTASH

This is a great recipe that I came up with for my pal Shaun, the guy who hates all vegetables except corn and edamame. This was a fun way to get some good stuff into him. It's quick, tasty, and will please your vegetarian friends as well as any vegetable-phobic people you have in your life.

SERVES 4

1 tablespoon butter, or more as needed

1 tablespoon CBD Olive Oil (page 7)

1 small onion, finely diced

1 small red pepper, seeded and finely diced

One 10-ounce box frozen corn, thawed (see Note)

One 12-ounce bag frozen shelled edamame (soybeans), thawed

Splash of chicken or vegetable stock

2 teaspoons CBD Salt (page 13)

Freshly ground black pepper

In a large sauté pan over medium heat, heat the butter and oil. Add the onion and pepper and cook until soft. Add the corn, edamame, and stock, stir, then partially cover and cook until the corn and soybeans are warmed through, 3 to 5 minutes. Add the salt and pepper to taste. Serve.

note

If you have beautiful, in-season sweet corn on the cob available, then cut the kernels off 4 to 5 ears and use those instead of the frozen corn.

ROASTED VEGETABLES

Roasted vegetables aren't just for fall and winter—depending on the season, almost any vegetable can be roasted this way, and they're good hot or cold.

4 medium red potatoes or 6 to 8 small new potatoes, cut into 2-inch cubes, parboiled for 10 minutes, and drained

4 carrots, peeled and cut into 1-inch pieces

1 onion, cut into large dice

2 red bell peppers, seeded and cut into 1-inch pieces

2 turnips or parsnips, peeled and cut into 1-inch pieces

3 to 4 garlic cloves, peeled

Salt and freshly ground black pepper

3 tablespoons CBD Olive Oil (page 7)

2 tablespoons CBD Butter (page 7), melted

Fresh lemon juice, oregano, and/or parsley, for garnish

Preheat the oven to 375°F. Line a large baking sheet with parchment paper.

In a large bowl, toss the vegetables with 2 teaspoons of salt, pepper to taste, and the oil. Spread the vegetables on the baking sheet. Roast for 1 hour, flipping a few times, and continue to cook until they pierce easily with a fork and are browned around the edges. Drizzle with the butter and a spritz of fresh lemon juice, sprinkle with herbs, and serve immediately.

MUSHROOMS *in* BRANDY CREAM

When I want to treat my best pal, Toni, I make her this and she loses her mind. These mushrooms are great over a beautiful steak, mashed potatoes, egg noodles, or anything that would welcome creamy mushroom goodness. They are even lovely on thick, toasted bread . . . try it and see!

SERVES 4

2   tablespoons butter

1   tablespoon CBD Butter (page 7)

1   pound cremini or white mushrooms, wiped clean and sliced

1   large shallot, finely diced

¼   cup brandy

½   cup heavy cream or half-and-half

Salt and freshly ground black pepper

Fresh Italian parsley leaves, for garnish

In a skillet over medium heat, gently melt the butters. Add the mushrooms to the pan in a single layer. Cook without moving them around until browned, 5 to 10 minutes. Add the shallot and stir to combine. Cook for a 2 to 3 minutes or until the shallot starts to turn translucent, then add the brandy and reduce the heat to low. After the smell of alcohol has subsided, turn off the heat and add the cream, stirring to combine. Return the heat to medium and cook briefly to heat through, then taste and adjust the seasoning with salt and pepper to taste. Garnish with parsley and serve hot.

AVGOLEMONO (GREEK EGG *and* LEMON SOUP)

This clean, simple Greek soup is wonderful; the lemon elevates it to a glorious place.

4   cups rich chicken stock (homemade if you have it)

¼   cup uncooked orzo or short-grain white rice

3   eggs

3   tablespoons lemon juice

1   teaspoon CBD Glycerin Tincture (page 10)

Salt

In a large saucepan, bring the stock to a boil, then add the orzo or rice. Reduce the heat and cook until tender, 6 to 7 minutes for orzo and about 10 if using rice. Reduce the heat to low and let sit while you prepare the eggs. In a medium bowl, whisk the eggs and lemon juice together until smooth. Ladle about 1 cup of the warm stock into the egg mixture and whisk to combine. Add the egg mixture to the saucepan and stir until the soup becomes cloudy and thickens, about 2 minutes. Stir in the tincture and salt to taste, and serve hot.

SPLIT PEA SOUP

This classic is inexpensive and endlessly variable, it will warm you up, and it feeds a lot of people. If you have the time, this soup is even better when you cook it with a big, meaty ham bone—it makes a deeply delicious soup, but it does take longer to get the flavor and the ham off the bone. To make this vegetarian, just omit the ham and use vegetable stock.

SERVES 6 GENEROUSLY

- 2 tablespoons olive oil
- 1 tablespoon CBD Olive Oil (page 7)
- 1 large white onion, chopped
- 1 large carrot, peeled and diced
- 2 ribs celery, diced

- 2 to 3 cloves garlic, minced
- 1 pound green split peas, picked over and rinsed
- 6 to 8 cups chicken stock
- 1 pound diced ham with some fat (optional)

- 1 ham bone (optional)
- 2 teaspoons CBD Glycerin Tincture (page 10)
  Salt
- 1 teaspoon red pepper flakes
- 1 teaspoon dried thyme

In a heavy stockpot over medium heat, heat the olive oils and add the onion, carrot, and celery. Cook until softened, about 10 minutes, then add the garlic and cook, stirring constantly, until fragrant, about 1 minute. Add the peas, stock, ham and ham bone if using, and bring to a boil. Reduce the heat, partially cover the pot, and let it simmer until the peas are soft, at least 30 minutes. (The longer you cook the soup, the thicker it gets, so keep an eye on it. If using a ham bone, plan on at least another hour of cooking and using the larger amount of stock.) When the consistency is to your liking, add the tincture and 1 teaspoon of salt (the saltiness of the soup will depend on your ham, so taste and adjust when the soup is done), red pepper flakes, and thyme. Serve hot in big bowls with some good bread on the side.

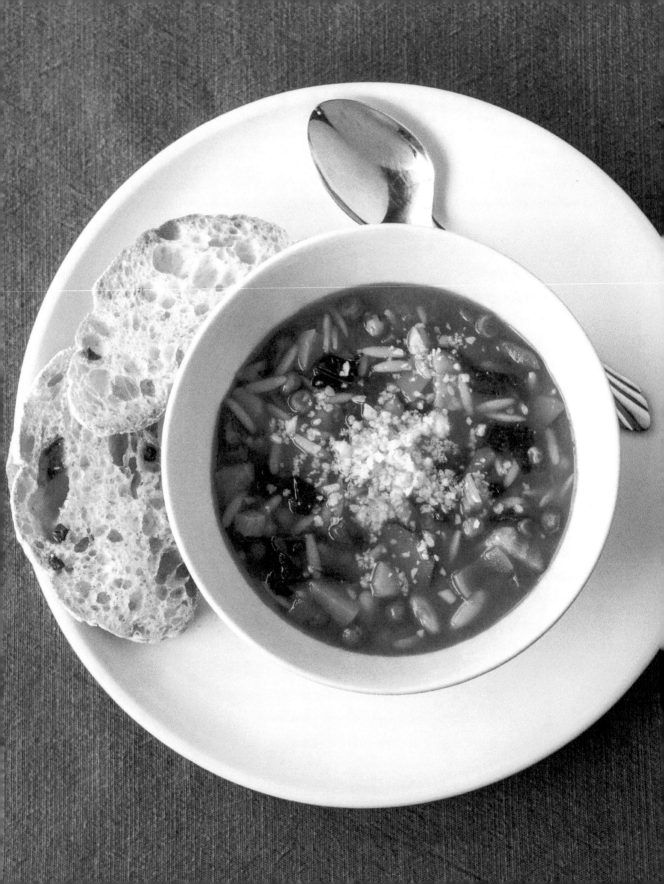

GREENEST MINESTRONE

This is one of those classics that is only improved by the addition of infused butter and oil. It's already minestrone heaven even before the CBD is introduced with a float of infused oil, pesto, or chimichurri before serving. This can easily be made vegan—just use vegetable broth and leave off the Parmesan.

2 to 3 tablespoons olive oil

1 large onion, chopped

2 carrots, peeled and diced

2 stalks celery, diced

2 tablespoons tomato paste

2 cups chopped firm seasonal vegetables (zucchini, summer squash, peas, green beans, etc.)

4 to 5 cloves garlic, minced

½ teaspoon dried thyme

½ teaspoon dried oregano

One 28-ounce can diced tomatoes

6 cups chicken or vegetable broth (or water)

Salt and freshly ground black pepper

Red pepper flakes

½ cup uncooked orzo or rice

One 15.5-ounce can white beans

(cannellini or navy work great)

2 cups chopped kale

2 tablespoons CBD Butter (page 7)

1 tablespoon CBD Olive Oil (page 7), CBD Basil Pesto (page 83) or CBD Chimichurri (page 27)

Lemon juice and freshly grated Parmesan, for garnish

In a large saucepan or Dutch oven over high heat, heat the olive oil. When it begins shimmering, add the onion, carrots, celery, and tomato paste. Reduce the heat to medium-low and cook, stirring occasionally, until the vegetables are soft and the tomato paste is darker in color, 8 to 10 minutes. Add the vegetables, garlic, and herbs and stir well to combine, then add the diced tomatoes and broth. Season with salt and pepper, and red pepper flakes to taste. Bring it just to a boil, then reduce the heat, partially cover the pot, and simmer for 15 minutes. Add the orzo or rice, beans, and kale, and cook until the orzo or rice is tender, about 10 minutes for orzo and 15 for rice. Just before serving, stir in the butter, float the CBD oil, pesto, or chimichurri on top, and sprinkle with lemon juice and Parmesan.

ENTRÉES

MAC 'N' CHEESE

This is a classic and has everything you want in macaroni and cheese—rich, creamy, comforting goodness, plus a crunchy, buttery breadcrumb topping.

SERVES 6

1 pound elbow macaroni

5 tablespoons butter, divided

1 medium onion, finely diced

3 tablespoons all-purpose flour (substitute 1 tablespoon CBD Flour [page 4] for all-purpose here if you like the taste)

Cayenne pepper

1 tablespoon dry mustard

3 cups milk, warmed

1 bay leaf

1 teaspoon paprika

1½ teaspoons CBD Salt (page 13), or to taste

½ teaspoon freshly ground black pepper

¾ pound (12 ounces) sharp cheddar, grated

1 cup chopped ham or pancetta (optional)

1 tablespoon CBD Butter (page 7)

1 cup panko breadcrumbs

4 ounces Gruyère, grated

Preheat the oven to 350°F. Cook the macaroni until al dente and drain. Meanwhile, in a saucepan over medium heat, melt 3 tablespoons of the butter. Add the onion and cook for 5 minutes or until translucent, then whisk in the flour, cayenne to taste, and mustard. Cook, stirring, for 5 minutes or until blended and light brown. Add the milk, bay leaf, and paprika, whisking to ensure there are no lumps. Add the salt and pepper, simmer for 10 minutes or until thick, then remove the bay leaf. Stir in three-quarters of the cheddar (8 ounces) and the ham if using, then fold in the macaroni and pour the mixture into a 3-quart casserole. In a small saucepan over medium-low heat, melt the remaining 2 tablespoons of butter and CBD butter, add the panko, and mix until coated. Top the macaroni mixture with the remaining cheddar, Gruyère, and the panko. Bake for 30 minutes or until the top is brown and bubbly. Let sit for 10 minutes before serving.

CLASSIC CHEESE SOUFFLÉ

This recipe is adapted from the great Julia Child, and
I think it's the epitome of cheesy goodness.

2 tablespoons finely grated Parmesan

1½ tablespoons butter

1 tablespoon CBD Butter (page 7)

3 tablespoons all-purpose flour

1 cup whole milk, warmed to steaming

½ teaspoon paprika

½ teaspoon CBD Salt (page 13)

Pinch of nutmeg

4 egg yolks

5 egg whites

1 cup grated Gruyère, packed

Preheat the oven to 400°F and position a rack in the lower part of the oven. Butter a 6-cup soufflé dish, add the Parmesan, and tilt the dish so the sides are coated with the cheese. In a large saucepan over medium heat, melt the butters. Add the flour and whisk until the mixture starts to foam, about 3 minutes, taking care not to let it brown. Remove from the heat and let it sit for about 1 minute. Add the warm milk, whisking until smooth. Return to the heat and cook, whisking constantly, until very thick, 2 to 3 minutes. Remove from the heat and stir in the paprika, salt, and nutmeg. Add the egg yolks, whisking to blend after each addition. Scrape the mixture into a large bowl and cool to lukewarm. In another bowl, beat the egg whites with a hand mixer until they're stiff but not dry. Fold about one-quarter of the egg whites into the egg yolk mixture to lighten it, then in two additions gently fold in the remaining whites. Carefully fold the Gruyère into the mixture, taking care to not deflate the egg whites. Transfer the batter to the prepared dish, place in the oven, and immediately turn the heat down to 375°F. Bake until puffed and golden brown and the center moves only slightly, about 25 minutes. Do not open the oven door during the first 20 minutes of baking. Serve immediately.

SAUSAGE FRITTATA

I've gone to this recipe again and again, and it never lets me down. And here's the glory of the frittata: you can serve it hot, room temperature, even cold and it's wonderful. It's a recipe that lets seasonal ingredients shine, so feel free to use whatever vegetables look freshest and best at the market. For a beautiful vegetarian brunch, lunch, or dinner, omit the sausage and substitute ½ cup of sliced mushrooms—or your favorite vegetable.

SERVES 4 TO 6

1 tablespoon olive oil

1 medium onion, chopped

2 sweet Italian sausages, casing removed and crumbled

1 small zucchini, diced

1 small red pepper, diced

CBD Salt (page 13) and freshly ground black pepper

1 cup leftover cold pasta or 1 cooked potato, chopped

6 large eggs, beaten

2 tablespoons CBD Butter (page 7), cold and cubed

½ cup freshly grated Parmesan, or more as needed

Preheat the oven to 350°F. In a large ovenproof sauté pan over medium low heat, warm the oil. Add the onion and cook until translucent, about 5 minutes. Add the sausages and cook until there's no pink remaining. Drain off most of the fat, then add the remaining vegetables and cook until soft, about 5 minutes. Taste and adjust seasoning with salt and pepper to taste. Add the pasta or potatoes to the pan, then pour in the eggs, resisting the urge to move them. Let them settle around the vegetables and sausage and cook until they're set on the bottom and around the edges, 5 to 7 minutes. When the eggs look mostly set, dot the top with the butter, then sprinkle with Parmesan. Put the pan in the oven and let it cook until the eggs are firm in the middle, 6 to 8 minutes. When everything is firm and the cheese is melted, remove from the oven and let it cool a bit, then slide onto a plate and cut into wedges. Season with more CBD salt to taste and serve.

ONE-PAN PASTA

This easy dish is the essence of summer and simplicity,
and adding CBD only makes it better.

1 pound linguine

1 pound cherry or grape tomatoes, cut in half

1 sweet onion, thinly sliced

4 to 6 cloves garlic, thinly sliced

2 to 3 sprigs basil, plus leaves for garnish

2 tablespoons olive oil, plus more for serving

1 tablespoon CBD Olive Oil (page 7)

1 teaspoon CBD Salt (page 13)

1 teaspoon red pepper flakes, or to taste

4½ cups water

Salt and freshly ground black pepper, to taste

Freshly grated Parmesan, for serving

Combine all of the ingredients except the Parmesan in a large, straight-sided skillet. Bring just to a boil, reduce the heat to low, and let simmer. Stir and turn the mixture with tongs until the pasta is al dente and the water has almost evaporated, about 9 minutes. Taste and adjust seasoning, sprinkle with Parmesan, and serve.

LEMON LINGUINE

This is one of those elegantly simple recipes that is way more than the sum of its parts; it's all about the best ingredients. Do get the best fresh pasta, the juiciest lemons, and the richest cream . . . you'll be very happy you did!

SERVES 4

1   pound fresh linguine (see Note)

¼   cup (2 ounces) unsalted European butter

1   teaspoon CBD Butter (page 7)

1   cup heavy cream

¼   cup fresh lemon juice

3   teaspoons lemon zest

2   teaspoons CBD Salt (page 13)

    Freshly ground black pepper

    Freshly grated Parmesan, for serving

Cook the pasta until al dente—fresh only takes a couple of minutes. Drain and reserve ½ cup of the cooking water. Meanwhile, in a large skillet over medium-low heat, melt the butters, then stir in the cream and lemon juice. Remove from the heat, cover, and keep warm. Add the pasta to the skillet with the lemon zest and 1 to 2 tablespoons of the reserved cooking water and mix well. Add more pasta water if it seems dry. Add salt and pepper to taste, top with lots of Parmesan, and serve.

note

You can use dried pasta instead of fresh. Fettucine and spaghetti also work well with this dish.

PASTA *with* FRESH TOMATO SAUCE

This is a great recipe to have on hand when you don't really want to cook, but you still want something good. You can use more or less olive oil, vinegar, and salt to your taste.

¾ cup good-quality olive oil

2 teaspoons CBD Olive Oil (page 7)

1½ tablespoons balsamic vinegar

1½ tablespoons red wine vinegar

3 to 4 pounds ripe tomatoes, cut into medium dice

Handful of basil or oregano leaves, chopped

¼ cup dried hemp bud, decarbed (see page 4) and very finely chopped

1 large clove garlic, minced

Salt and freshly ground black pepper

1 pound spiral pasta (like fusilli or rotini)

In a large bowl, mix the oils and vinegars, then add the tomatoes, squishing them to release some juice. Stir in the herbs and hemp, then add garlic and salt and pepper to taste. Cover the bowl and let marinate at room temperature for about an hour. Cook the pasta until al dente and drain. Add the pasta to the tomato mixture, and let stand for 15 minutes at room temperature. Taste, adjust seasoning with salt and pepper to taste, and serve.

3P PASTA (PESTO, PEAS, *and* PARMESAN)

This is simple, inexpensive, and really tasty; fresh peas and fragrant basil will guarantee you a fine meal. If you'd like to make this vegan, leave out the Parmesan from the pesto and the pasta.

SERVES 4

1 pound pasta (shells, or any small, cup-shaped pasta)

1 cup fresh peas (you can also use frozen and thawed)

1 cup CBD Basil Pesto (page 83)

CBD Salt (page 13) and freshly ground black pepper

Freshly grated Parmesan, for garnish

Chopped fresh basil leaves, for garnish

Cook the pasta until al dente. Drain, reserving ½ cup of the cooking water. Working quickly, put the hot pasta in a big serving bowl and add the peas. Mix in ½ cup of the pesto, taste, and add salt and pepper to taste. If it seems dry, add 1 to 2 tablespoons of the reserved pasta water and a bit more pesto. Sprinkle with the Parmesan and basil and serve.

CBD BASIL PESTO

1   cup fresh basil leaves
½   cup pine nuts, toasted
½   cup freshly grated Parmesan
2   cloves garlic, peeled
2   teaspoons lemon zest
1   teaspoon CBD Salt (page 13), or to taste
1   teaspoon red pepper flakes, or to taste
2   tablespoons olive oil
1   tablespoon CBD Olive Oil (page 7)

Put all of the ingredients except the oils in a food processor and process until chunky. With the machine running, slowly pour in the oils and blend until it's the desired consistency. Taste and adjust the seasoning. Serve over almost any protein, or with vegetables, pasta (as above), or crostini.

PUMPKIN PENNE

This is a great fall dish, lovely as a side dish or as an entrée. To make it vegan, replace the cream with vegetable stock, coconut cream, or nut cream.

SERVES 4

1 pound penne pasta

1 tablespoon olive oil

1 large onion, chopped

1 large red pepper, chopped

2 to 3 cloves garlic, minced

1 cup dry white wine, like Pinot Grigio

½ cup vegetable or chicken broth

1 cup canned pumpkin

1 to 2 fresh sage leaves, minced

2 teaspoons CBD Salt (page 13)

Freshly ground black pepper

1 teaspoon cinnamon

¼ teaspoon nutmeg

½ cup heavy cream or half-and-half

2 to 4 tablespoons Sage or Autumn Spice CBD Butter (page 15), melted

Freshly grated Parmesan and minced sage leaves, for garnish (optional)

Cook the pasta until al dente and drain. Meanwhile, in a skillet over medium heat, warm the olive oil and add the onion and red pepper. Sauté until softened, 7 to 8 minutes, then add garlic and stir for about 1 minute, or until fragrant. Add the wine and cook, uncovered, until the liquid is reduced to about half. Add the broth, pumpkin, sage, salt, pepper to taste, cinnamon, and nutmeg. Add the cream and heat through, then add the drained pasta to the sauce and stir to coat. Drizzle with CBD butter, top with Parmesan and sage if using, and serve.

PORK POTSTICKERS

These are so very delicious you might never buy them again; homemade is so much better.
You can also make them ahead of time and freeze for a delicious meal anytime (see Note).

MAKES 36

DIPPING SAUCE

- 3 tablespoons soy sauce
- 1 teaspoon CBD Glycerin Tincture (page 10)
- 2 teaspoons rice wine vinegar

POTSTICKERS

- 1 pound ground pork
- 1 teaspoon CBD Oil (page 7), preferably vegetable or peanut
- 1 cup shredded green cabbage tossed with 1 tablespoon salt and drained in a colander for 30 minutes
- 3 ounces shiitake mushrooms, diced
- 2 cloves garlic, minced
- 2 green onions, thinly sliced
- 1 tablespoon hoisin sauce
- 1 tablespoon freshly grated ginger
- 2 teaspoons sesame oil
- 1 teaspoon sriracha, or to taste
- ¼ teaspoon white pepper
- 36 wonton wrappers
- 2 tablespoons vegetable oil

MAKE THE DIPPING SAUCE: In a small bowl, mix together all the ingredients and set aside.

MAKE THE POTSTICKERS: In a large bowl, combine pork, CBD oil, cabbage, mushrooms, garlic, green onions, hoisin, ginger, sesame oil, sriracha, and white pepper.

To assemble the dumplings, place wrappers on a work surface. Spoon 1 tablespoon of the pork mixture into the center of each wrapper. Using your finger, rub the edges of the wrappers with water. Fold the dough over the filling to create a half-moon shape and pinch the edges to seal.

In a large skillet over medium heat, warm the vegetable oil. Add 2 tablespoons of water and the potstickers in a single layer, cook covered for 2 minutes, then uncover to crisp—you'll need to do this in batches). Serve immediately with dipping sauce.

note

To freeze, place uncooked potstickers in a single layer on a parchment-lined baking sheet overnight. Transfer to freezer bags. These will keep up to three months in the freezer. Cook from frozen as above, but you'll need to add a few minutes to the covered cook time to heat through.

KALE AND SAUSAGE STEW

This is an easy stew that tastes great, comes together quickly, and fills you up. It's super-healthy, especially with the addition of CBD. For a great vegan version, leave out the sausage and Parmesan and use vegetable stock.

SERVES 6

- 2 tablespoons olive oil
- 1 large onion, diced
- 1 red pepper, seeded and diced
- 2 stalks celery, diced
- 1 large carrot, peeled and diced
- 12 ounces andouille or Italian sausage, sliced

- 1 bunch kale, stemmed and chopped
- Salt and freshly ground black pepper
- 3 to 4 cloves garlic, minced
- 1 quart rich chicken or vegetable stock
- One 14-ounce can diced tomatoes with juice

- One 14-ounce can white beans, drained and rinsed
- 2 teaspoons CBD Glycerin Tincture (page 10)
- Red pepper flakes
- Freshly grated Parmesan (optional)

In a large skillet over medium-high heat, warm the olive oil. Add the onion, pepper, celery, carrot, and sausage, and cook, stirring, until onion is just tender, about 10 minutes. Drain off about half of the fat, then reduce the heat to medium-low. Add kale, 2 teaspoons salt, and garlic; cover and continue cooking for 2 minutes; again, you don't want to the garlic to brown. Add the chicken stock, tomatoes with juice, white beans, and tincture and stir. Taste and adjust seasoning, cover, and cook for 15 to 20 minutes, or until the vegetables are tender. Taste and adjust seasoning with pepper flakes and pepper to taste, sprinkle with Parmesan if using, and serve in large bowls with crusty bread.

LUSCIOUS LENTIL STEW

Lentils are a great pantry staple; they can be made into all kinds of dishes and, unlike other legumes, cook in about 30 minutes. For this stew, get dependable green or brown lentils; the orange, red, or black ones will cook too quickly. For a vegetarian version, leave out the sausages.

SERVES 4

2 to 3   tablespoons olive oil

1   medium onion, chopped

1   small carrot, peeled and diced

1   stalk celery, diced

2 to 3   fresh sweet Italian sausage links, sliced (optional)

1 to 2   cloves garlic, minced

1   tablespoon tomato paste

1½   cups dry lentils

4½   cups stock, broth, or water

4 to 5   kale leaves, stemmed and chopped (optional)

Salt, pepper, dried oregano, and red pepper flakes, to taste

Splash of red wine vinegar

1   tablespoon CBD Olive Oil (page 7)

2 to 3   tablespoons chopped fresh parsley, for garnish

In a large saucepan or Dutch oven over medium heat, warm the olive oil. Add the onion, carrot, and celery and cook until they start to soften, about 10 minutes. Add the sausages, and reduce the heat to medium low. Cook, stirring, until the sausages are almost done and no longer pink, then add the garlic and cook about 1 minute, until fragrant. Stir in the tomato paste, lentils, and stock. Turn up the heat and bring just to a boil, then reduce the heat. Simmer gently until the lentils are soft, 20 to 30 minutes (start checking early; overcooked lentils can get mushy). Toward the end of the cooking time, add the kale and cook for 2 to 3 minutes. When the lentils are done, add the seasonings to taste, and stir in the vinegar and the CBD oil. Depending on the stock you use, you might need up to 1 teaspoon more salt, so taste and adjust seasoning as needed. Garnish with the parsley and serve in big bowls with crusty bread for dipping.

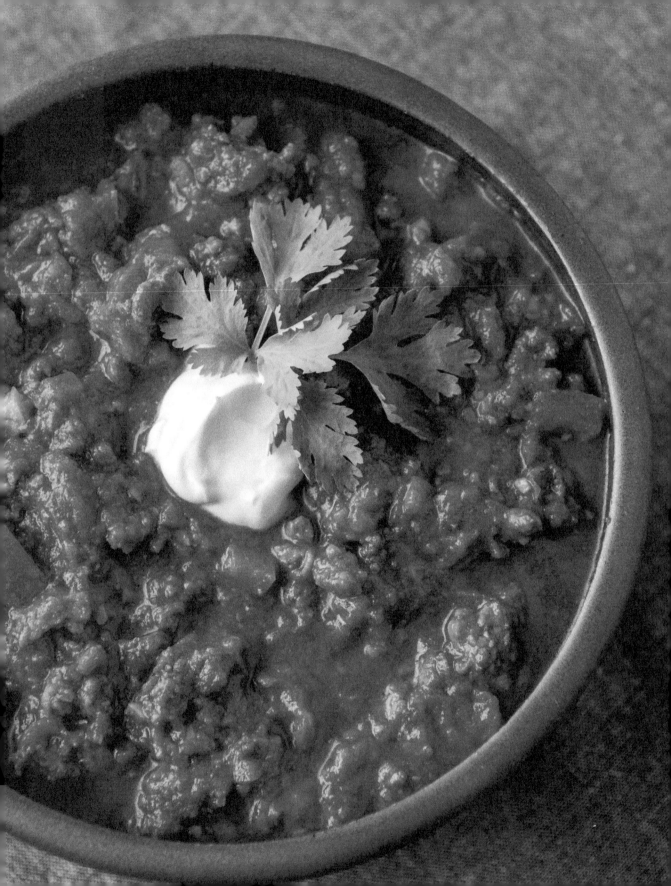

NO-BEAN CHILI

Usually I like to use stew-type meats like chuck for chili, but with the addition of CBD butter and CBD oil, it's necessary to cook for less time. Using ground beef makes this quick and CBD-friendly.

SERVES 4 TO 6

1 pound lean ground beef (90/10 or 85/15)

½ pound ground pork or ground turkey (dark meat is best)

1 large onion, chopped

1 red or yellow pepper, seeded and diced

3 to 4 cloves garlic, minced

One 28-ounce can crushed tomatoes

2 tablespoons chili powder

1 tablespoon chipotle chili powder or smoked paprika

1 tablespoon CBD Butter (page 7)

1 tablespoon CBD Glycerin Tincture (page 10)

Salt and freshly ground black pepper

1 tablespoon red wine vinegar

Chopped fresh oregano, sour cream, cotija cheese, and/or chopped cilantro, for garnish

In a large saucepan or Dutch oven over medium heat, add the ground beef and pork. Cook, breaking up the meat, then add the onion and pepper. Cook, stirring frequently, until the meat starts to brown and the onion is translucent, 8 to 10 minutes. Add the garlic, cook for about 1 minute until fragrant, then add the tomatoes, chili powders, butter, tincture, and salt and pepper to taste. Bring this just to a boil, then reduce the heat to low and simmer, partially covered, 30 to 45 minutes. Sprinkle with the vinegar, garnish with oregano, sour cream, cheese, and cilantro, and serve.

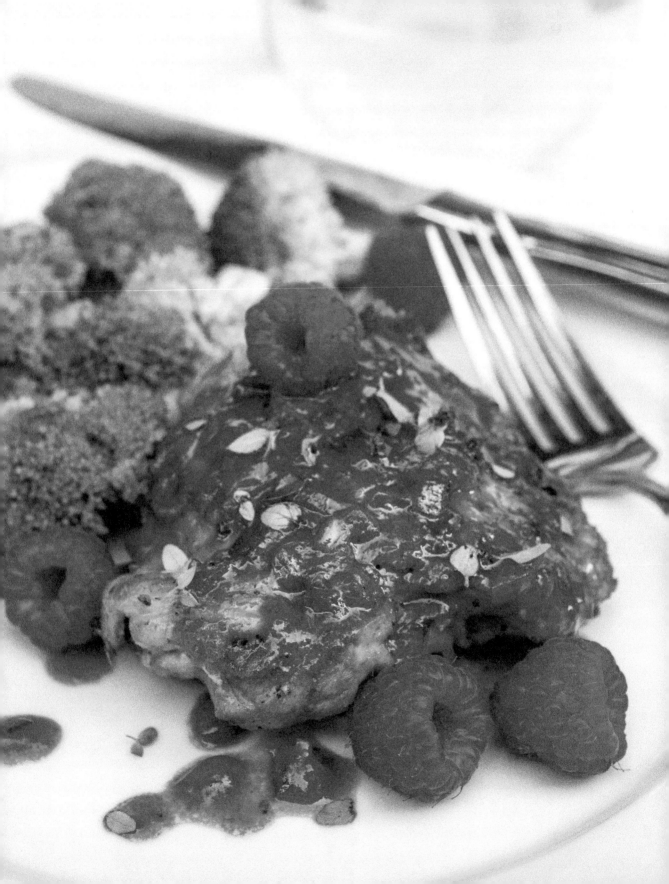

CHICKEN *with* RASPBERRIES

Fresh raspberries and thyme perfume this dish with the scent of summer. It's wonderful alongside a light green salad, preferably served al fresco on a warm, breezy evening.

SERVES 4

1½ cup fresh raspberries, divided

4 large chicken thighs or breasts (see Note)

Salt and freshly ground black pepper

1 tablespoon butter

1 tablespoon olive oil

2 tablespoons fresh thyme leaves, ½ minced and ½ whole, divided

½ cup dry white wine

2 tablespoons white balsamic vinegar

½ small white onion or 1 large shallot, minced

½ cup chicken stock

2 tablespoons CBD Butter (page 7)

Push half of the raspberries through a sieve to make a purée and set aside. Season the chicken well with salt and pepper. In a large skillet over medium-high heat, melt the butter with the oil. When the butter stops foaming, add the chicken skin side down and let it cook for a few minutes. Reduce the heat to medium and cook until the skin is brown (about 5 minutes), then turn it. Scatter half the whole thyme leaves over the chicken, reduce heat to medium-low, cover, and cook until the chicken is cooked through, or a meat thermometer reads 165°F, about 20 minutes. Remove the chicken and keep warm in a low oven. Discard the fat from the skillet and add the wine, vinegar, onion, and minced thyme and deglaze the pan for 2 minutes, scraping up any delicious brown bits. Add the stock and boil until it's reduced by half. Reduce the heat to low, stir in the reserved raspberry purée, add the CBD butter, and warm through. Slice the chicken or leave it whole and serve with a drizzle of the pan sauce, a sprinkle of thyme leaves, and the remaining whole berries scattered over.

note

This dish works great with either breasts or thighs; just make sure you get bone-in and skin-on local chicken for maximum flavor. If you have time, salt the chicken well and let it sit in the fridge, covered, overnight—dry brining equals guaranteed moistness.

GINGER CHICKEN

I came up with this recipe when I had a lot of ginger in the house and it's quite delightful, especially when served over steamed jasmine rice.

4 to 6 bone-in, skin-on chicken thighs, patted dry

2 tablespoons CBD Olive Oil (page 7)

1 small onion or 1 large shallot, thinly sliced

2 large carrots, peeled and sliced

5 cloves garlic, minced

3 to 4 tablespoons finely minced or grated fresh ginger

1 tablespoon candied ginger, minced

½ cup dry white wine

¼ cup soy sauce

Spicy Sweet CBD Butter (page 14), melted (optional)

Sliced green onion, sesame seeds, and pickled ginger, for garnish

Preheat the oven to 325°F. Place a large ovenproof skillet over medium-low heat and add the thighs, skin side down. Cook 12 to 15 minutes or until the skin turns brown and they release easily from the pan. (As the skillet heats up, the chicken will gradually release fat, so there's no need to oil the skillet. Don't be tempted to rush this, and resist the urge to move them around in the pan; they'll let go when they're ready.) Remove the thighs to a plate. Drain off the chicken fat, reduce the heat to low, and add the CBD oil. Add the onion and cook, until starting to look translucent, about 5 minutes. Add the carrots, garlic, and fresh and candied ginger, and stir. Add the wine, and deglaze the pan, scraping to release any browned bits. When the smell of the wine has cooked off, add the soy sauce and return the chicken to the pan, skin side up. Cover, move to the oven, and bake for 45 minutes. Meanwhile, five minutes before the end of cooking, preheat the broiler. Uncover the pan and put it under the broiler—not too close—for about 5 minutes, or until the skin is beautifully brown. Drizzle with the CBD butter if using, garnish with the green onion, sesame, and ginger, and serve hot over rice.

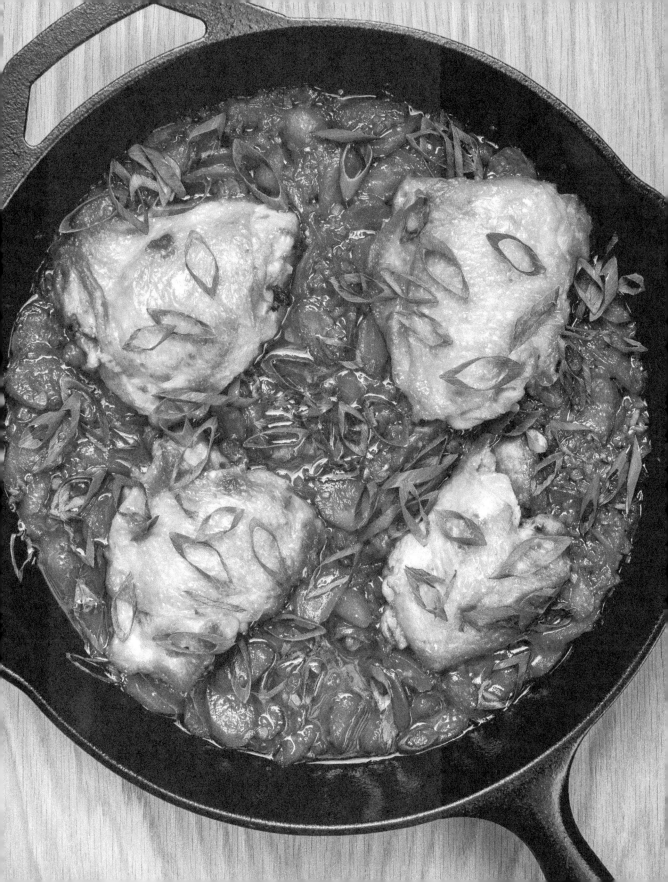

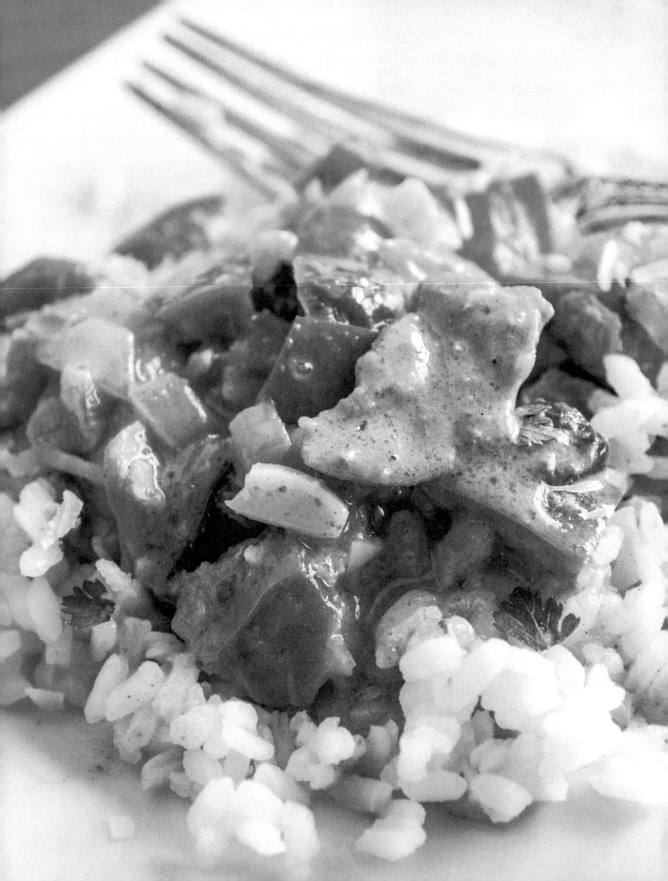

COCONUT CHICKEN CURRY

This recipe gives you a great curry; you can stretch it with additional broth, spice it up with some chili sauce, or otherwise customize it to suit your taste buds.

SERVES 4

- 2 tablespoons CBD Oil (page 7), preferably canola or peanut
- 1 large white onion, chopped
- 1 large carrot, peeled and diced
- 2 to 3 cloves garlic, minced
- 1 tablespoon all-purpose flour

- 3 to 4 tablespoons curry powder, or to taste
- 1 tablespoon garam masala
- 1 pound boneless skinless chicken thighs, cubed
- 1 can coconut milk
- ½ cup chicken broth
- ½ cup golden raisins, soaked in warm water and drained

- 1 teaspoon CBD Salt (page 13)
- 1 tomato, seeded and diced
- 2 tablespoons CBD Butter (page 7)

Shredded coconut, mango chutney, and roasted peanuts for garnish

In a large saucepan or Dutch oven over medium heat, heat the oil. Add the onion and carrot and cook until the onion is soft and translucent, about 10 minutes, then add the garlic and cook, stirring, for about 1 minute, or until fragrant. Sprinkle with the flour, curry powder, and garam masala. Reduce the heat to low and cook until the vegetables start to brown, 6 to 8 minutes. Raise the heat to medium-low, add the chicken, mix well, and let cook about 10 minutes. Add the coconut milk, broth, and raisins and stir while the sauce thickens, about 10 minutes. When it's thick and the chicken is no longer pink, add the salt, taste and adjust the seasoning, and add the tomatoes and the CBD butter and stir them in. Cook until warmed through, remove from the heat, and let cool slightly. Garnish with the coconut, chutney, and peanuts and serve hot over cooked rice.

LARB GAI

This is a classic Thai salad—easy, quick, and always delightful as an entrée. Spooning into the lettuce leaf cups to eat makes for a fun and enjoyable meal. If you can, use ground dark meat for the chicken—it has a higher fat content, which you'll want for this recipe.

SERVES 4 TO 6

- ⅔ cup fresh lime juice
- ⅓ cup fish sauce (nam pla or similar)
- 1 tablespoon sugar
- 2 teaspoons Thai roasted chili paste in oil or chili-garlic sauce
- 1 tablespoon CBD Oil (page 7), preferably vegetable or peanut
- ¾ cup chicken broth
- 1½ pounds ground chicken (preferably dark meat)
- 1 cup thinly sliced green onions
- ¾ cup thinly sliced shallots
- 3 tablespoons minced fresh lemongrass
- 1 tablespoon thinly sliced Thai chilies or serrano chiles
- ½ cup chopped fresh cilantro leaves
- ⅓ cup chopped fresh mint leaves
- Salt and freshly ground black pepper
- 2 small heads Boston lettuce, separated into leaves

In a medium bowl, whisk the lime juice, fish sauce, sugar, chili paste, and oil to combine; set aside. In a large, heavy skillet over medium heat, bring the broth to a simmer. Add the chicken and simmer, breaking up the meat with a spoon, until cooked through, 6 to 8 minutes. Add the green onions, shallots, lemongrass, and chilies. Cook, stirring, until the vegetables are tender and most of liquid has evaporated, about 4 minutes. Remove from the heat. Stir in the reserved sauce, cilantro, and mint. Taste and season with salt and pepper to taste. Serve spooned into or wrapped up in the lettuce leaves.

GROUND BEEF STROGANOFF

This recipe uses only six main ingredients and is surprisingly delicious, proving once again that simplicity can be perfection.

SERVES 4

1 tablespoon CBD Olive Oil (page 7)

1 tablespoon olive oil

1 large onion, thinly sliced

1 pound 80/20 ground beef

2 to 3 tablespoons all-purpose flour

1 cup beef stock, preferably homemade

2 teaspoons CBD Salt (page 13)

Freshly ground black pepper

1 cup sour cream

In a large skillet over medium-low heat, heat the oils and add the onion. Cook until soft. Add the ground beef and cook, stirring, until it's broken up and no longer pink. Sprinkle with the flour and cook, stirring, 2 to 3 minutes until everything is coated with flour, then add the beef stock and stir in. Taste and adjust the seasoning, adding the salt and pepper to taste. Simmer until thickened. Just before serving, remove from the heat and stir in the sour cream; don't let it cook or the cream will separate. Serve hot over rice, egg noodles, or hearty toasted bread.

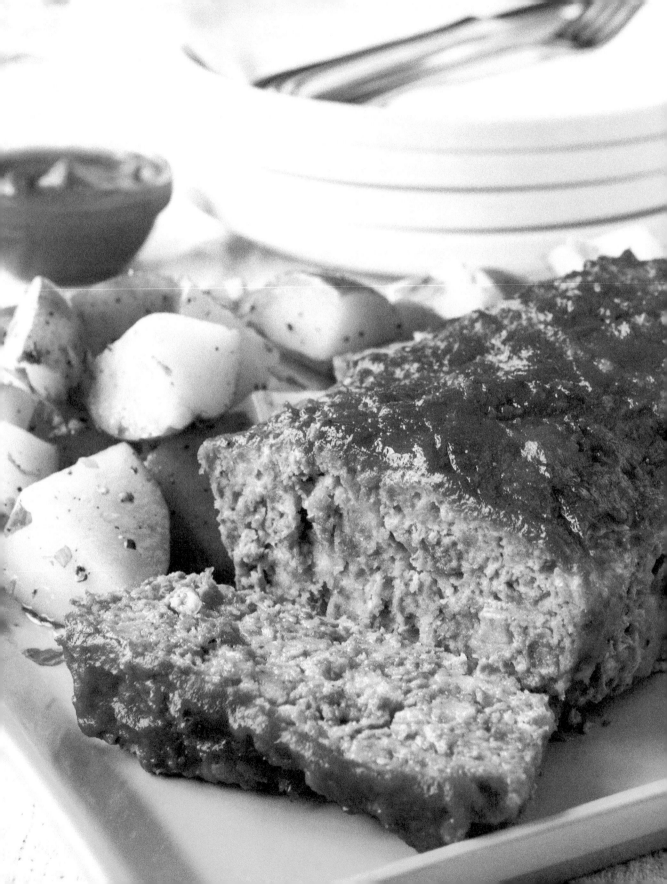

MAGIC MEATLOAF

Fabulous as a meatloaf, this mixture can also be used for a multitude of other tasty dishes—meatballs (see Variation) and burgers, for example. When topped with CBD Ketchup (page 17) and CBD Spicy Mustard (page 19) or served alongside garlic bread (page 42) and a crisp salad with CBD Vinaigrette (page 29), this will guarantee a very happy evening.

SERVES 4 TO 6

- 1 pound ground beef (80/20)
- ½ pound ground pork sausage
- 2 eggs, beaten
- 2 cloves garlic, minced
- ½ cup plain dry breadcrumbs or panko
- ¼ cup milk or half-and-half
- ½ small onion, finely diced
- 1 tablespoon CBD Glycerin Tincture (page 10)
- 2 tablespoons CBD Butter (page 7), softened
- Salt and freshly ground black pepper
- 2 teaspoons dried oregano or marjoram
- Meatloaf Glaze (recipe follows)

Preheat the oven to 350°F. In a large bowl, combine the beef and sausage—wet hands work best here. Add the eggs and garlic. In a small bowl, mix the breadcrumbs with the milk, then add to the meat mixture, along with the onion, tincture, butter, salt and pepper to taste, and oregano. Mix to incorporate.

Pat the mixture into a loaf pan and bake for 1 hour, or until the top is brown and the fat has cooked out. Meanwhile, if you would like to glaze the meatloaf, prepare the glaze. Remove the meatloaf after 45 minutes in the oven, spread the glaze over the top, and return to the oven for 5 to 10 minutes, or until the glaze has browned. Drain the fat and discard. Cool slightly on a rack, slice, and serve warm.

continues on the next page

MEATLOAF GLAZE

- 2 tablespoons CBD Ketchup (page 17)
- 1 tablespoon CBD Spicy Mustard (page 19)
- 1 tablespoon brown sugar

In a small bowl, mix all the ingredients to combine.

VARIATION

To make meatballs, form the mixture into balls the size of a golf ball, then simmer in your favorite marinara sauce for at least 20 minutes, or bake them in a parchment-lined baking sheet at 375°F for 20 minutes. You could also shape them into teeny cocktail meatballs: Fry till cooked through, and serve with toothpicks and dipping sauce.

LAMB STIR-FRY

This is a great way to use lamb; I adapted this from *Bon Appétit*, and it cooks fast and tastes fancy.

SERVES 4

1 pound boneless leg of lamb, thinly sliced against the grain

4 to 5 garlic cloves, minced

2 tablespoons CBD Olive Oil (page 7)

1 tablespoon red wine vinegar

2 teaspoons ground cumin

1 teaspoon ground coriander

1 teaspoon paprika

Salt and freshly ground black pepper

2 tablespoons olive oil

1 red onion, cut into wedges

½ cup plain full-fat Greek yogurt

2 teaspoons CBD Salt (page 13), or more to taste

Freshly ground black pepper

½ cup pomegranate seeds

Chopped pistachios, chopped mint, and chopped parsley, for garnish

In a medium bowl, toss the sliced lamb with the garlic, CBD oil, vinegar, cumin, coriander, and paprika. Season with salt and pepper to taste, and chill for about 15 minutes. In a large skillet over medium-high heat, warm the 2 tablespoons of olive oil. Add the lamb and cook in batches so it browns nicely, about 4 minutes per batch, then set aside. In the same skillet, add the onion and cook for about 3 minutes, stirring, until it starts to soften. Add ½ cup water and cook and stir a bit more until the water evaporates, about 3 minutes. Return the lamb to the skillet and toss it with the onion. Stir in the yogurt, then adjust the seasoning with salt and pepper to taste. Sprinkle on the pomegranate seeds, garnish with pistachios, mint, and parsley, and serve over rice or alongside warm, toasted pita bread.

FISH IN PARCHMENT

This is inspired by a French dish, fish *en papillóte*. It's essentially fish baked in parchment or foil with flavorings and vegetables. It's very easy and delicious, as well as an impressive dinner party dish: There's a dramatic reveal when guests open their packet of steamy deliciousness. You can really use almost any kind of vegetable, as long as they cook in the same time as the fish.

SERVES 4

½ large onion, thinly sliced

2 carrots or 1 small red pepper, cut into julienne

½ pound thin green beans, trimmed and sliced on the diagonal into thirds

Four 6-ounce fish fillets (almost any kind will work)

½ cup dry white wine

¼ cup CBD Olive Oil (page 7), for drizzling

2 teaspoons CBD Salt (page 13)

Freshly ground black pepper

Lemon zest and chopped parsley, for garnish

Preheat the oven to 375°F. Cut 4 pieces of parchment paper or foil large enough to hold a fish fillet and vegetables without leaking when folded in half. Layer the vegetables and fish on the paper and sprinkle with the wine, oil, salt, and pepper to taste. Crimp the edges, then place the packets on a sheet pan and bake until the fish is cooked through and the vegetables are soft, about 15 minutes, depending on the thickness of the fish. Serve the packets immediately on individual plates (but it's worth warning guests about the steam that will emerge!).

PARMESAN-CRUSTED HALIBUT

I adapted this recipe from one I found years ago in the *Seattle Times*. The creamy, golden Parmesan crust works beautifully with the firm yet tender halibut fillets. It's dreamy when served with a bright green salad or grilled asparagus with a squeeze of lemon.

SERVES 4

FOR THE CRUST

- ¼ cup mayonnaise
- 2 teaspoons fresh lemon juice
- 2 small garlic cloves, finely minced
- 1 teaspoon CBD Spicy Mustard (page 19)
- 2 tablespoons freshly grated Parmesan
- 1 green onion, finely chopped
- Dash of hot sauce

FOR THE HALIBUT

- Four 4-to-6-ounce halibut fillets
- 2 teaspoons fresh lemon juice
- Freshly ground black pepper
- 2 teaspoons CBD Salt (page 13)

FOR THE CRUST: In a small bowl, combine all of the ingredients and set aside.

FOR THE HALIBUT: Preheat the oven to 450°F. Put the fish on a broiler pan and sprinkle with the lemon juice, and pepper to taste. Bake for 10 minutes per inch of thickness, about 15 minutes total, or until the white flesh is just starting to flake. Remove from the oven and turn on the broiler. Sprinkle the fillets with salt and spread on the crust mixture. Place under the broiler, and broil for 1 minute or until the topping is golden. Serve immediately.

SPANISH FISH

This is a great way to get a lot of flavor from the more inexpensive types of white fish; I like snapper, but whatever is fresh at the fish store will do. Feel free to substitute 1 teaspoon turmeric for the saffron. You'll miss out on the subtle, complex flavor of the saffron, but the turmeric gives the dish the same golden yellow hue for a fraction of the price.

SERVES 4

- 1 tablespoon olive oil
- 1 tablespoon CBD Olive Oil (page 7)
- 1 large white onion, chopped
- 2 to 3 cloves garlic, chopped
- One 28-ounce can tomato sauce

- 1 tablespoon cumin
- Large pinch of saffron
- ½ cup golden raisins
- Large pinch red pepper flakes, or to taste
- 2 teaspoons CBD Glycerin Tincture (page 10)

- Four 6-ounce white fish fillets
- 12 large pimiento-stuffed green olives, sliced
- 2 teaspoons CBD Salt (page 13)
- Freshly ground black pepper

In a large skillet over medium heat, warm the olive oils. Add the onion and sauté until translucent, about 5 minutes. Add the garlic and cook for about 1 minute, or until fragrant. Add the tomato sauce, stir, then add the cumin, saffron, raisins, pepper flakes, and tincture and stir. Reduce heat to low and simmer for at least 10 minutes, or up to an hour on super-low heat; the goal is a beautiful, thick tomato sauce. When you're ready to serve, bury the fish fillets in the sauce, sprinkle on the olives, cover the pan, and cook on medium to medium-low heat for about 10 minutes, or until the fish is cooked through. Taste and adjust the seasoning with the salt and pepper to taste. Serve with rice and a good light red wine.

DESSERTS

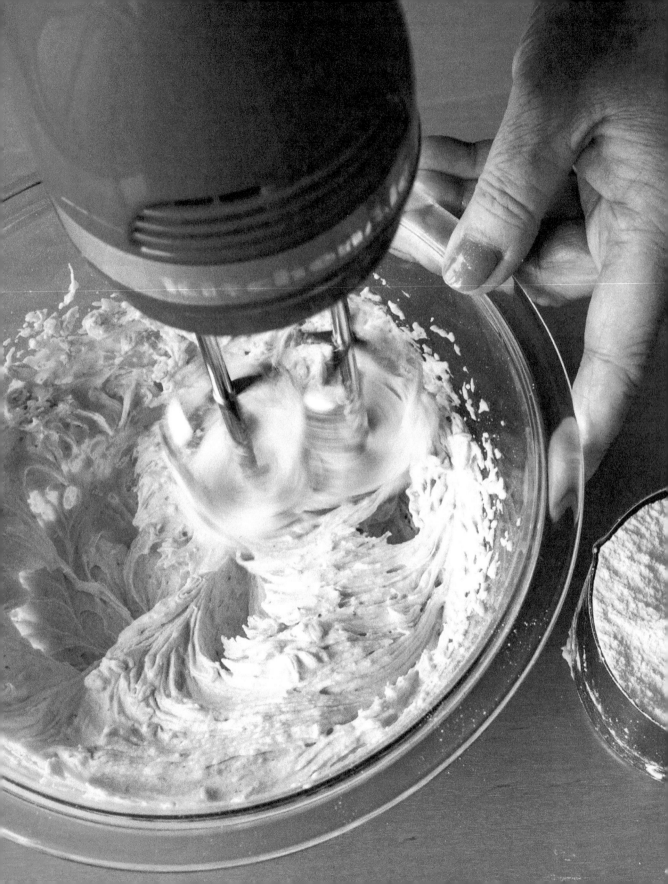

CBD BUTTERCREAM FROSTING

This rich frosting will take your baked goods to the next level—the CBD butter guarantees it! Feel free to play around with it—use orange instead of lemon, stir in some chopped nuts, or add food coloring. The flavors are up to you. This recipe makes enough to frost a layer cake or 2 dozen cupcakes.

MAKES 3 CUPS

2½ cups powdered sugar

½ cup CBD Butter (page 7)

½ cup unsalted butter

1 teaspoon vanilla extract

1 to 2 tablespoons heavy cream (adjust amount for the thickness you prefer)

Zest and juice of 1 lemon

In the bowl of a stand mixer, combine the sugar and butters and beat on low speed, then turn it up and mix for three more minutes. Add the vanilla, cream, lemon zest, and a little of the lemon juice and beat for another minute or so. Taste and adjust the tartness and the consistency to your taste with the more cream or juice.

POM CLOUDS

This cloudlike parfait is my favorite kind of dessert—simple, delicious, elegant, and not that bad for you. Pomegranate seeds have a lot of vitamins and make it festive and pretty. If you use ginger cookies, try extra dark chocolate; with the almond cookies, you might like a milk chocolate.

SERVES 1

3 to 4 thin almond or ginger cookies, crushed

½ cup CBD Whipped Cream (recipe follows)

Best-quality dark chocolate, for garnish

Pomegranate seeds, for garnish

Put the crushed cookies in the bottom of a nice glass and cover with some of the whipped cream. Shave as much chocolate as you like over it and sprinkle with pomegranate seeds; repeat the layers, ending with a sprinkle of seeds.

CBD WHIPPED CREAM

1	cup heavy cream
2 to 3	grams CBD Flour (page 4)
1	tablespoons powdered or granulated sugar

Put the heavy cream in the top of a double boiler. Add the CBD Flour. Let this cook slowly over low heat, 30 minutes to 1 hour. Strain the infused cream through a cheesecloth set in a sieve, then let cool completely. Store in a glass container in the fridge until ready to use. When ready to whip, put the cold cream in a chilled bowl (the colder the better, as this ensures good whipping). Add the sugar and beat until soft peaks form. Leftover unwhipped cream is delicious in your coffee.

FROZEN BERRIES *with* HOT WHITE CHOCOLATE

A love letter to summer berries—blueberries, blackberries, raspberries, strawberries—this recipe lets their beautiful flavor shine, isn't too heavy, and is great for brunch or after dinner. Enjoy with port, rosé, bubbly, or whatever makes you happy.

SERVES 8

1 pound best-quality white chocolate, chopped

2 cups heavy cream

2 tablespoons vanilla extract

1 teaspoon CBD Glycerin Tincture (page 10)

CBD Salt (page 13), to taste

2 pounds fresh berries, cleaned and frozen (or use frozen berries)

Combine the chocolate, cream, vanilla, tincture, and salt in a double boiler and melt over simmering water, stirring until blended. About 10 minutes before serving, divide frozen berries among individual bowls, then drizzle the hot sauce over the berries.

ADULT APPLESAUCE

This is a great fall dessert and can be tailored to your tastes with sweetened whipped cream, chopped nuts, crushed cookies—whatever you like; it's also good as a side with roast pork or chicken.

6 to 8 apples (Fuji, Honeycrisp, and Gala are good), cored and cubed

1 cup red wine (Merlot, Lemberger, Pinot Noir, or Syrah)

½ cup grade B pure maple syrup

2 cinnamon sticks

¼ teaspoon salt

¼ teaspoon ground cloves

¼ teaspoon red pepper flakes or chili powder

2 teaspoons CBD Glycerin Tincture (page 10)

Whipped cream, chopped nuts, or crushed cookies for garnish (optional)

In a large stockpot over low heat, place the apples, wine, syrup, and spices. Cook until reduced to the desired consistency. If you prefer a more sauce-like consistency, mash with a potato masher. Remove from the heat, remove the cinnamon sticks, and stir in the tincture. Let cool and serve. Store in a glass container in the fridge.

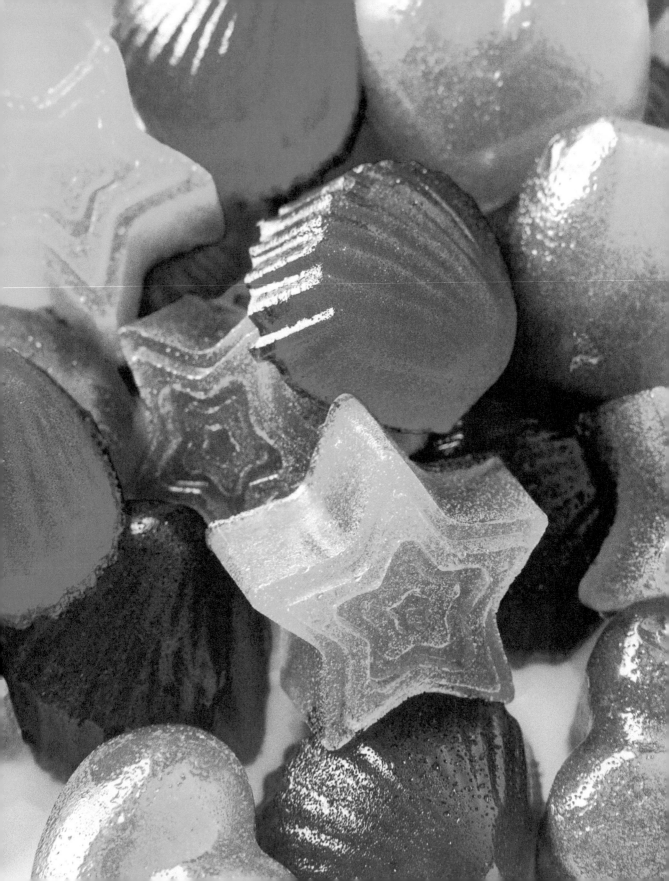

GROWN-UP GUMMIES

Gummies can be a fine way to get your medicine; they're simple to make and fun to eat, and are a perfect little bite whenever you need some relief. The main caution here is kids: if there are any littles around, make sure they can't get in to these—they are very tempting. You'll need some special equipment (a funnel or dropper and silicone gummy molds, available online) for these treats, so be sure to get everything ready before you begin.

MAKES ABOUT 30, DEPENDING ON SIZE OF MOLDS

Nonstick cooking spray

1 large packet (6 ounces) Jell-O, your preferred flavor

Four ¼-ounce envelopes unflavored gelatin

½ cup cold water

¼ cup CBD Alcohol Tincture (page 10)

Cornstarch, for dusting

Special equipment: silicone gummy molds, funnel or dropper

Grease the molds lightly with the cooking spray, then wipe with a paper towel so very little oil remains. Place the molds on a rimmed baking sheet. In a small saucepan, whisk the Jell-O and gelatin together, then add the cold water and whisk to combine. Over medium heat, bring Jell-O mixture to a boil, then reduce heat to low and cook for 5 minutes, stirring often. Remove from the heat and let cool slightly. Add the tincture and mix well. Using a funnel or dropper, fill the molds. Place the baking sheet in the fridge and let chill for 15 minutes. Pop the gummies out of the molds and dust lightly with cornstarch to prevent sticking. Store in a glass container in the fridge.

CRUNCHY NUT-BUTTER CUPS

If you loooooove peanut butter cups as much as I do, you're going to have a great time with these. They're like a layered, high-end peanut butter cup, but with added crunch and CBD. You'll fall in love with these frozen treats!

MAKES 24 MINI CUPS

1 cup unsalted toasted almonds

1 cup pitted dates

2 tablespoons cocoa powder

1 tablespoon CBD Butter (page 7)

½ cup peanut or cashew butter

1 tablespoon almond flour

½ cup semisweet chocolate chips, melted

2 tablespoons CBD Oil, any kind (page 7)

½ teaspoon almond extract

1 teaspoon vanilla extract

Sparkling sugar, for finishing

Line a 24-cup mini muffin tin with muffin papers. In a food processor, combine the almonds, dates, cocoa powder, and CBD butter and pulse until it holds together. Press about 1 tablespoon of the almond mixture into the bottom of each cupcake liner. In a small bowl, combine the peanut butter and almond flour. Spread about 1 teaspoon of the peanut butter mixture on top of each cup. Place the tin in the freezer until the peanut mixture is firm. Meanwhile, in a small bowl, mix the chocolate chips, oil, and extracts. Remove the tin from the freezer and carefully spoon about 1½ teaspoons of the chocolate over each cup and smooth to the edges. Sprinkle with the sparkling sugar, freeze until firm, and enjoy. Store cups in an airtight container in the freezer.

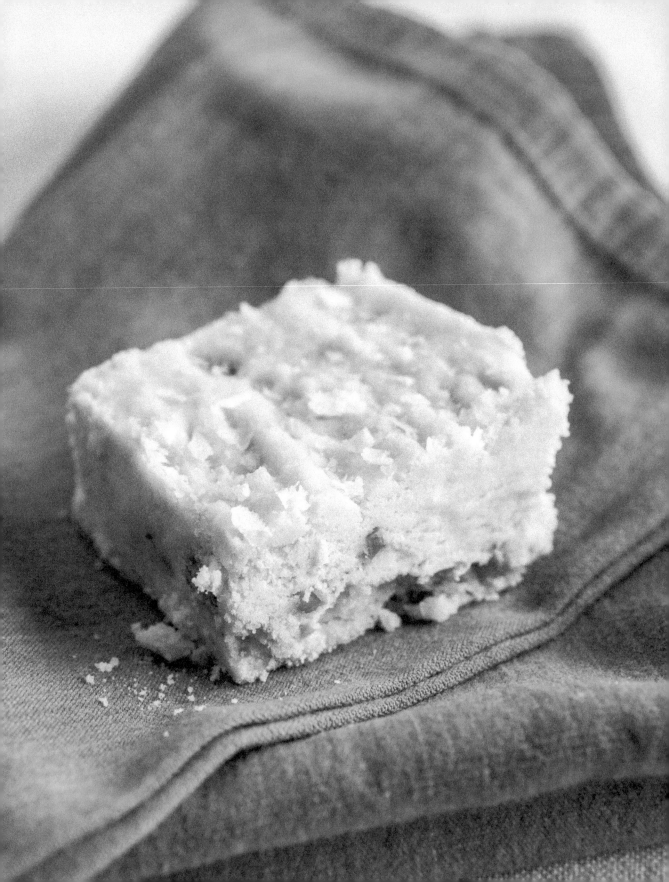

SEA SALT SHORTBREAD

I adapted this recipe from one in the good old *Joy of Cooking*—these are easy, buttery, and totally delicious!

MAKES ABOUT 24

1 cup CBD Butter (page 7; see Note)

½ cup sifted powdered sugar

2 cups sifted all-purpose or whole-wheat pastry flour

Pinch of salt

Zest of 1 large lemon

Maldon or another flaky sea salt, for finishing

Preheat the oven to 325°F. Line the bottom of a 9×13-inch baking pan with parchment paper (see Note). In a medium bowl, cream the butter with a hand mixer until it's very light, then add the sugar and beat until incorporated. Blend in the flour. Pat the dough into the pan evenly. Prick the dough all over with a fork. Bake for 45 to 50 minutes, or until golden, then sprinkle lightly with the flaky salt while still warm. When completely cool, remove from the pan and cut into 1½-inch squares.

notes

You can use half CBD Butter and half unsalted butter if you prefer.

You can vary the pan size according to your preferences: use a 9-inch square pan for thick cookies or a 9×13-inch for thinner ones.

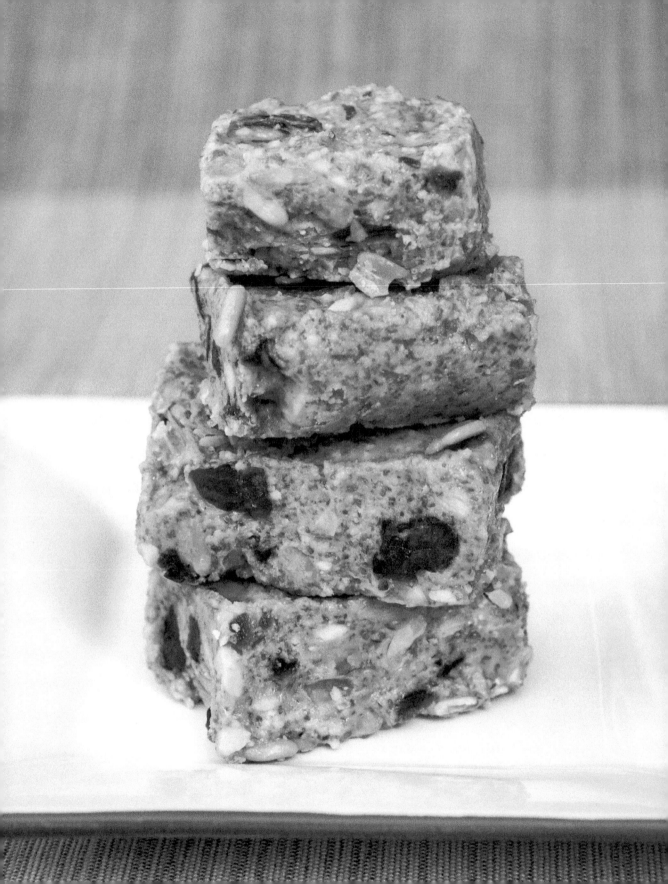

PEANUT BUTTER FUDGE BALLS

Tasty, nutritious, and easy to make, this is a delightful combination that makes wonderful (and effective!) fudge. Feel free to make substitutions: dried cranberries instead of raisins, or almond butter instead of peanut butter, or roll in cocoa powder and powdered sugar instead of chocolate chips. One thing is for sure: these won't last long!

MAKES ABOUT 36

1 cup natural peanut butter, drained of oil

6 to 8 tablespoons CBD Butter (page 7)

1 cup almond meal, or more as needed

½ cup soaked and drained raisins (even better if you soak them in port)

½ cup flaked coconut and/or sunflower seeds

½ cup mini chocolate chips

Agave syrup or honey, to taste

In a medium bowl, combine the peanut butter and the butter, and mix until incorporated. Add the remaining ingredients and mix to incorporate. If mixture seems too gooey, add a bit more almond flour, a tablespoon at a time till it is the desired texture. Using clean, slightly moist hands, form the mixture into balls about 1 tablespoon each. Place on a parchment-lined baking sheet and chill in the fridge until they're firm. Store in a glass container in the fridge.

note
You can also press the mixture into a square and cut into bars.

THE BEST BROWNIES

I adapted these beauties from the Baker's chocolate recipe. They are truly simple to make and exceptionally delicious! The smoked chili powder adds a wonderful flavor dimension.

Nonstick cooking spray

4 ounces unsweetened baking chocolate, roughly chopped

1 cups CBD Butter (page 7; see Note)

2 cups sugar

1 teaspoon vanilla

3 eggs

1 cup all-purpose flour

1 cup pecans or almonds, toasted and chopped

1 tablespoon smoked chili powder, or to taste

Preheat the oven to 350°F and line a 9×13-inch pan with foil or parchment paper, overlapping the edges. Spray the foil with cooking spray and set aside. In a large glass bowl, place the chocolate and butter. Microwave in 30-second increments to keep from scorching the chocolate, about 2 minutes total. Stir in the sugar and let cool for a few minutes. Blend in the vanilla and eggs. Fold in flour, nuts, and chili powder, then spread evenly into the prepared pan. Bake 30 to 35 minutes, or until a toothpick comes out with fudgy crumbs clinging to it. Let cool completely in the pan. Use the foil to lift out and cut into 1½-inch squares.

note

You can use half CBD Butter and half unsalted butter if you prefer.

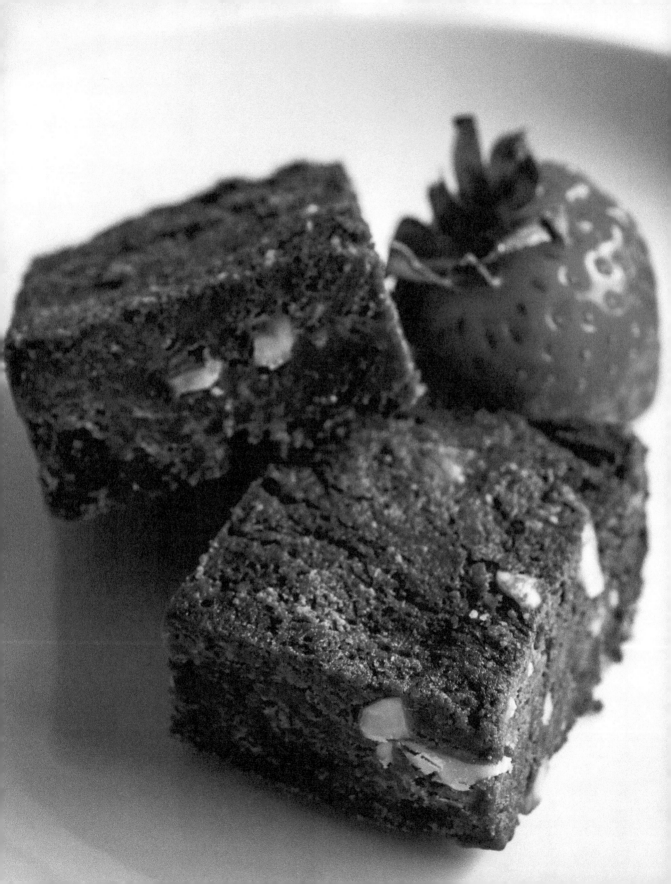

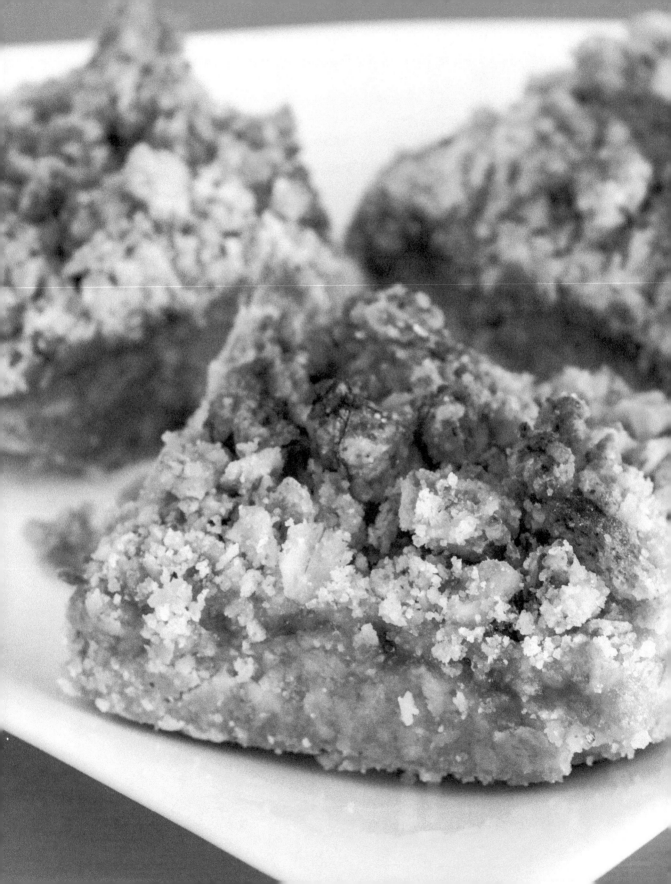

OATMEAL SQUARES

These are ridiculously easy to make and totally addictive. The hearty oats and sweet jam also make these the ideal breakfast bar. You can change up the jam filling and use the nuts or not—it's totally up to you.

MAKES ABOUT 16

1¼ cups old-fashioned rolled oats

1¼ cups all-purpose flour

½ cup finely chopped toasted walnuts (see Note)

½ cup sugar

½ teaspoon baking soda

¼ teaspoon salt

1 cup CBD Butter (page 7), melted

2 teaspoons vanilla

1 cup good-quality jam

4 whole graham crackers (8 squares), crushed

Whipped cream, for serving (optional)

Preheat the oven to 350°F. Grease a 9-inch square baking pan. In a large bowl, combine the oats, flour, walnuts, sugar, baking soda, and salt. In a small bowl, combine the butter and vanilla. Add the butter mixture to the oat mixture and mix until crumbly. Reserve 1 cup for topping, and press the remaining oat mixture into the bottom of the baking pan. Spread the jam evenly over the top. Add the crushed crackers to the reserved oat mixture and sprinkle over the jam. Bake for 25 to 30 minutes, or until the edges are browned. Cool completely in the pan on a rack. Cut into 16 squares. Serve, adding a dollop of whipped cream if desired. Store in a glass container in the fridge.

note
If you omit the nuts, increase the amount of flour by ¼ cup.

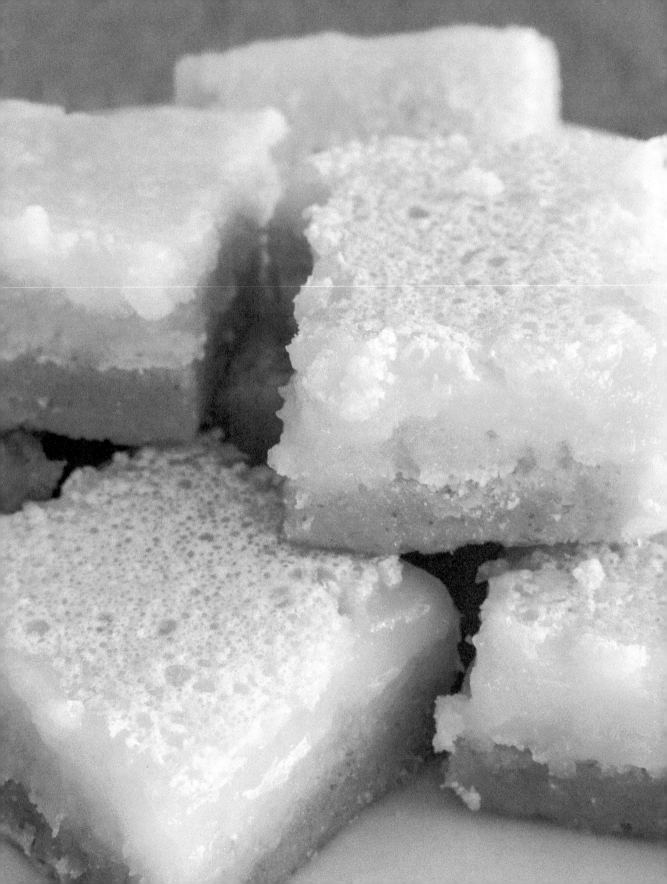

GLORIOUS LEMON BARS

This classic dessert is tart and puckery fun.

¼ cup CBD Butter (page 7), softened

½ cup butter, softened

⅔ cup powdered sugar, plus more for dusting

1½ cups plus 3 tablespoons flour, divided

2 tablespoons lemon zest

3 large eggs, slightly beaten

1¼ cups sugar

¼ cup fresh lemon juice

Preheat the oven to 350°F and grease a 9-inch square baking pan. In a large bowl, beat together the butters and sugar until blended. Fold in 1½ cups of the flour and the lemon zest until incorporated. Press the dough evenly into the bottom of the baking pan and prick it all over with a fork so it doesn't bubble up. Bake for 20 minutes or until golden. Meanwhile, in a small bowl, whisk the eggs, sugar, lemon juice, and the 3 tablespoons of flour until light and foamy. Pour this over the baked crust, then return to the oven and bake for 20 to 25 minutes or until the filling is just set. Cool, then dust with powdered sugar and cut into 24 bars.

ORANGE ALMOND CAKE

This showstopper looks and tastes decadent, and it's super easy to make. Oh, it's also gluten free and Paleo friendly! You can substitute lemons for the orange and blueberries for the raspberries.

2 cups packed almond flour, plus more for dusting

1 teaspoon baking powder

½ teaspoon baking soda

1 teaspoon ground cinnamon

1 teaspoon ground ginger

½ teaspoon salt

3 eggs, lightly beaten

⅔ cup honey plus 1 teaspoon, divided

¼ cup CBD Oil (page 7)

Zest and juice (¼ cup) of 1 orange

1 cup fresh raspberries

Whipped cream, chopped toasted almonds or pistachios, and powdered sugar, for garnish

Preheat the oven to 325°F. Grease a 9-inch springform pan and dust the inside with almond flour. In a large bowl, whisk together the almond flour, baking powder, baking soda, cinnamon, ginger, and salt. In another bowl, whisk together the eggs, ⅔ cup of the honey, oil, and orange zest. Add the egg mixture to the dry ingredients and fold in until just a few lumps remain, then gently fold in the raspberries. Scrape into the prepared pan and smooth the top. Bake for 45 to 50 minutes, or until the edges are browned and the center is set. Warm the remaining 1 teaspoon honey with the orange juice. Brush this onto the warm cake—it'll sink right in—then let it cool completely in the pan. To serve, garnish slices with whipped cream, chopped almonds or pistachios, and a dusting of powdered sugar.

note

You can also make this into 12 cupcakes. Bake about 20 minutes or until the edges are browned and the center is set. Brush on the honey glaze and let cool. Frost with CBD Buttercream Frosting (page 107).

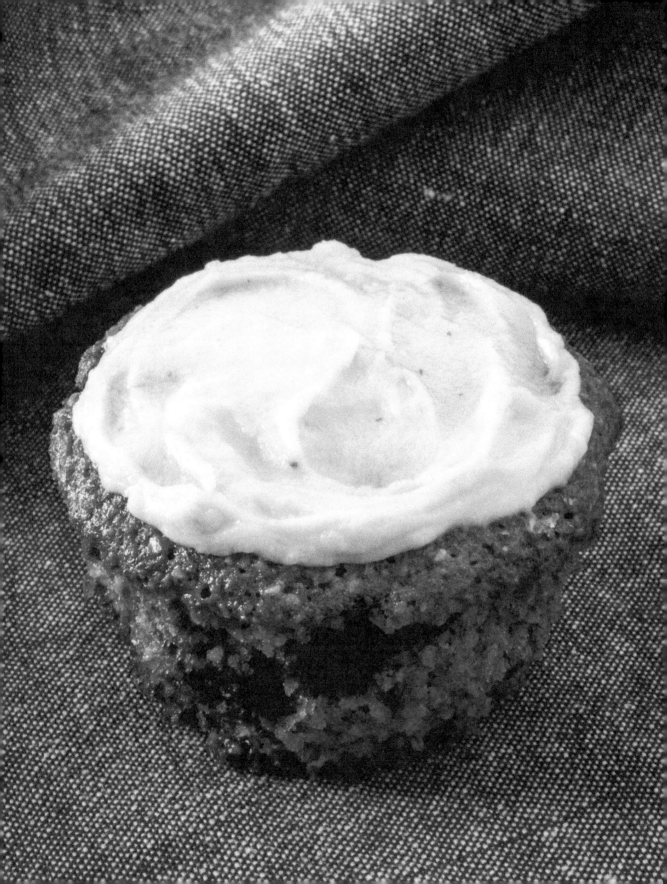

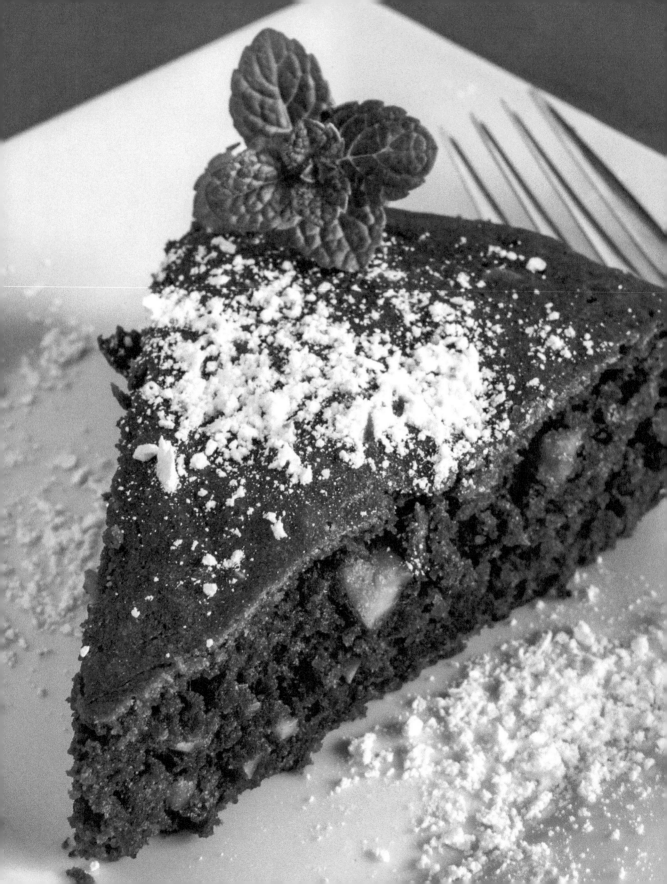

CHOCOLATE OLIVE OIL CAKE

This is a great recipe for medicated (and unmedicated) enjoyment. It's also vegan friendly, as there are no eggs or butter, just chocolatey goodness!

MAKES TWO 8-INCH LAYERS OR 12 BIG CUPCAKES

3 cups all-purpose flour

2 cups sugar

6 tablespoons good-quality cocoa powder

2 teaspoons baking soda

1 teaspoon salt

½ cup finely chopped nuts or dried fruit (optional)

¾ cup CBD Olive Oil (page 7)

2 tablespoons white vinegar

1 tablespoon vanilla

2 cups cold water

Powdered sugar, for dusting

Preheat the oven to 350°F. Grease and flour two 8-inch cake pans or line a 12-cup muffin tin with muffin liners. In a large bowl, combine the flour, sugar, cocoa powder, baking soda, salt, and nuts or dried fruit (if using). Whisk to incorporate. In another bowl, whisk together the oil, vinegar, vanilla, and water, then add to the flour mixture. With a hand mixer on medium-low speed, mix just until smooth. Pour into the prepared cake pans or muffin tin. Bake 30 to 40 minutes for cake or 20 to 25 minutes for muffins, or until a toothpick inserted in the center comes out clean (start checking early to avoid overbaking). Cool completely. Before serving, dust with powdered sugar.

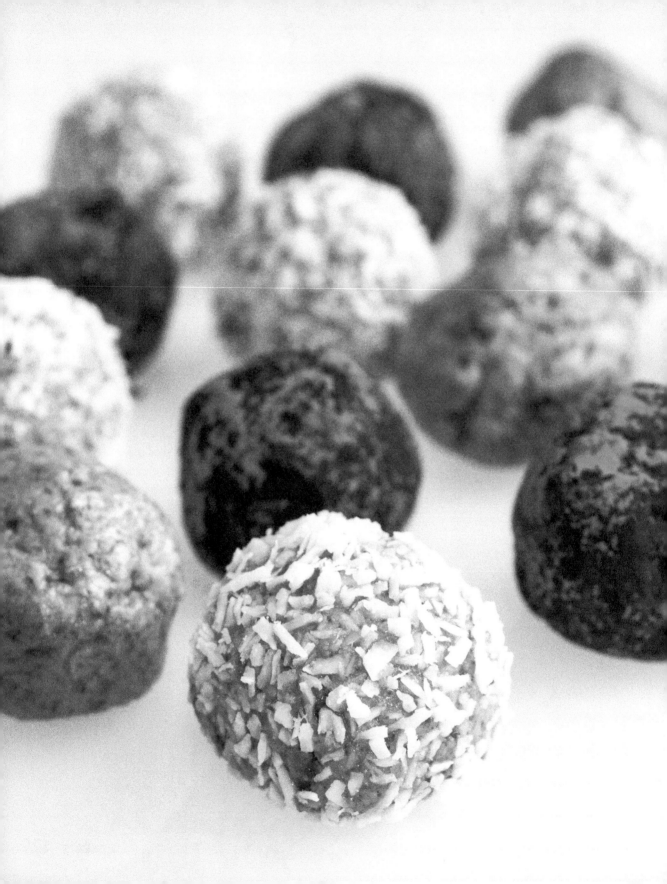

CHOCOLATE TRUFFLE BALLS

Super easy and remarkably delicious, these bite-sized wonders are a fine way to get your CBD! Adding whole almonds to the center gives these truffles a delightful, toothsome crunch. Remember to always store your CBD treats in the fridge and keep them away from the kids.

½ cup CBD Butter (page 7), softened

½ cup powdered sugar

¼ cup unsweetened cocoa powder

½ cup almond flour (see Note)

Large pinch salt

Dash almond extract

Dash vanilla extract

24 whole almonds, toasted in CBD Butter and CBD Salt (page 13; optional)

1 cup unsweetened shredded coconut

Line a baking sheet with parchment paper. In a medium bowl, combine all the ingredients except the whole almonds and coconut and mix gently until the mixture is fairly smooth. Roll teaspoons of the mixture between your palms into balls. (Work quickly, as the butter gets very soft quickly. Refrigerate for a few minutes if the mixture gets too soft.) If using the toasted almonds, tuck one into the center of each and roll again quickly to smooth things over. Place the coconut in a bowl and roll the balls in the coconut until coated. Place on the baking sheet, and refrigerate to firm up. Store in a glass container in the fridge.

note

You can substitute oat flour for the almond flour if you like.

GRILLED PEACHES *with* CINNAMON CREAM

When peaches are in season it's a wonderful thing. This recipe highlights their amazing taste and texture—the pure, luscious taste of summer—and the toppings are an extra-delicious bonus. Use all of them or only the ones you like. Any leftover mascarpone mixture is wonderful on toast, other fruits, or eaten late at night in front of the fridge.

SERVES 4 TO 8

2 pounds ripe peaches, halved and pitted

2 tablespoons canola oil

One 8-ounce container mascarpone cheese

1 teaspoon cinnamon, plus more to taste

2 teaspoons CBD Glycerin Tincture (page 10)

1 teaspoon vanilla

6 almond or gingersnap cookies, crumbled

¼ cup toasted almonds, finely chopped

Preheat the grill to high. (You can also do this on the stovetop in a cast iron skillet.) Brush the cut side of the peaches with the oil. Grill for 2 minutes cut side down, then flip and grill for another 3 to 4 minutes, until heated through. Meanwhile, in a small bowl, mix the mascarpone with the cinnamon, tincture, and vanilla. When the peaches are done, place them on a serving platter, fill with the spiced mascarpone, and garnish with the cookies, nuts, and a sprinkle of cinnamon.

CARROT MUFFINS

Carrot muffins are lovely for breakfast, a snack, or dessert—especially when topped with a cream cheese frosting.

MAKES 2 DOZEN

1¾ cups flour

1 teaspoon CBD Salt (page 13)

1 teaspoon cinnamon

1 teaspoon ground ginger

½ teaspoon grated nutmeg

¼ teaspoon baking soda

⅛ teaspoon baking powder

1 cup maple syrup

½ cup solid CBD Coconut Oil (page 7), melted, or ¼ cup CBD Oil mixed with ¼ cup vegetable oil

½ cup milk

1 tablespoon fresh lemon juice

1 teaspoon vanilla extract

2 cups grated carrot

½ cup crushed pineapple, drained

½ cup each raisins, coconut, and pecans (or any nuts you like)

Preheat the oven to 350°F. Line two 12-cup muffin tins with muffin papers or grease and flour the tins. In a large bowl, combine the flour, salt, cinnamon, ginger, nutmeg, baking soda, and baking powder. In a separate bowl, combine the maple syrup, coconut oil, milk, lemon juice, and vanilla. Add the wet ingredients to the dry and fold gently until just combined (overmixing makes the muffins tough). Fold in the carrots, pineapple, raisins, coconut, and pecans. Fill the prepared muffin tins two-thirds full. Bake for 25 to 30 minutes or until a toothpick inserted into the center of a muffin comes out clean. Let them cool a little before serving.

PEACH PIE

This glorious pie recipe is from my friend Julie, a baking goddess, who swears by using potato starch to thicken the fruit filling. It's a bit of work, but the results are incredible. Sub in nectarines for the peaches if you don't want to peel fruit. Get ready to serve to a large round of applause.

MAKES ONE 9-INCH PIE

½ cup plus 2 tablespoons CBD Sugar (page 12), divided

¼ cup packed brown sugar

5 cups fresh peaches, peeled and sliced (see Note)

1 CBD Double Pie Crust (recipe follows)

3 tablespoons potato starch or cornstarch

1 teaspoon cinnamon, divided

½ teaspoon ground cloves

¼ teaspoons CBD Salt (page 13)

1 tablespoon CBD Butter (page 7)

2 teaspoons lemon juice

3 tablespoons heavy cream

Preheat the oven to 400°F. In a large bowl, combine ½ cup of the CBD sugar and the brown sugar, add the peaches, and toss to coat. Cover and let stand for 1 hour. Roll out half of the chilled pie dough and lay it in the bottom of a 9-inch pie pan. Trim the edges, leaving about ½ inch of crust overhang. Drain the peaches, reserving the juice. In a small saucepan, combine the potato starch, ½ teaspoon of the cinnamon, the cloves, and CBD salt, and slowly add in the reserved peach juice and stir. Put the pan over medium heat, and bring to a boil. Cook for 2 minutes, or until thickened. Remove from the heat and stir in the CBD butter and lemon juice. Pour the mixture over the peaches, carefully fold in, then pour the filling into the crust. Roll out the remaining pastry and make a lattice or your favorite top crust. Trim, seal, and flute the edges. Mix together the remaining ½ teaspoon of cinnamon and 2 tablespoons CBD sugar. Brush the top of the uncooked pie crust with the cream and sprinkle with the cinnamon-sugar mixture. Cover the edges with foil so they don't bake too quickly, and bake for 50 to 60 minutes, or until the filling is bubbly and the crust is golden.

note
If you use frozen peaches, add 1 tablespoon more potato starch to the filling.

CBD DOUBLE PIE CRUST

3	cups all-purpose flour
14	tablespoons cold butter, cubed
2	tablespoons granulated sugar
2	tablespoons CBD Butter (page 7), cold
1½	teaspoons CBD Salt (page 13)
½	cup plus 2 teaspoons ice-cold water

Combine all of the ingredients except the water in the food processor. Pulse 4 to 5 times, then add the water, processing just until the dough comes together—you still want to see pea-size pieces of butter. Divide the dough into two equal pieces, wrap in plastic, and refrigerate for at least 1 hour or until ready to use.

MY MAJOUN

Majoun is a wonderful Moroccan confection of dried fruits, nuts, spices . . . and in this version, CBD. I found that the original recipe was too sweet for me—too many dates—so I put my own spin on it. This gooey dessert can be formed into balls and rolled in cocoa powder, used as a spread, or eaten from a spoon.

MAKES ABOUT 2 CUPS

1½ cups dried fruit, chopped—I like a mix of dates, raisins, and apricots, ½ cup of each

1 cup honey

½ cup ground toasted walnuts (hazelnuts and pistachios also work well)

½ cup ground toasted almonds

¼ cup water

1 teaspoon nutmeg

1 teaspoon aniseed

1 teaspoon ginger

2 to 3 tablespoons CBD Flour (page 4)

2 tablespoons CBD butter (page 7)

In a skillet, combine all of the ingredients except the CBD flour and butter and heat over low heat, stirring and smashing. When it's fully combined, pour into a glass container and stir in the CBD flour and butter. Store in the fridge.

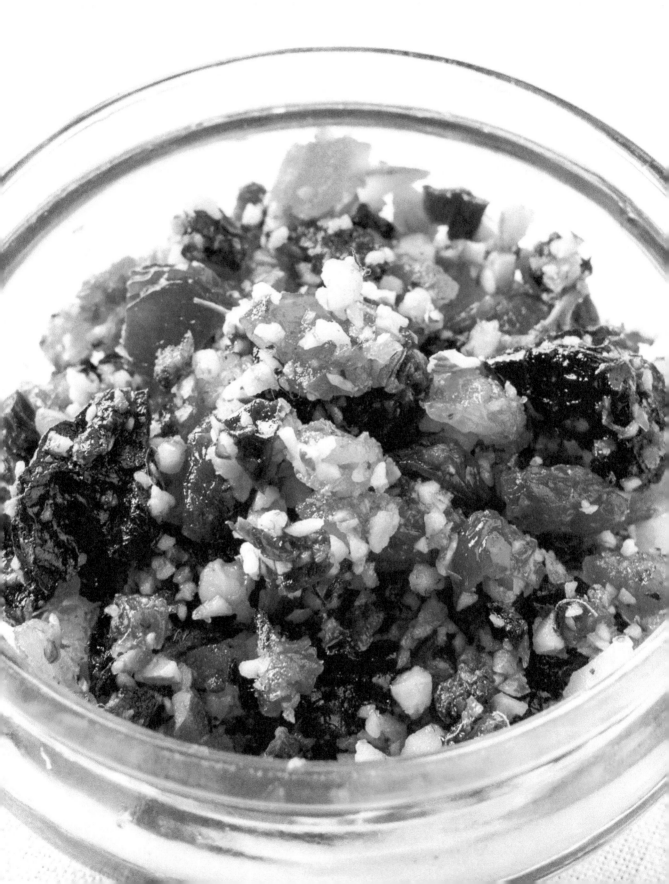

DESSERT TOAST

I come back to this easy dessert again and again, as it's amazingly simple but an absolute crowd-pleaser. You and your friends will be very happy, and even happier if you enjoy this with some port!

SERVES 4

Eight ¼-inch-thick baguette slices

1 tablespoon CBD Oil (page 7) mixed with 2 tablespoons olive oil

Eight 1-ounce squares best-quality dark chocolate

CBD Salt (page 13), for finishing

Preheat the oven to 350°F. Place the bread on a baking sheet and lightly brush each slice with the olive oil mixture. Place in the oven and bake until golden. Remove from the oven and put a square of the chocolate on each piece of bread, then return to the oven until the chocolate just starts to melt, just a minute or two. (You don't want the chocolate to seep through the bread.) Sprinkle salt on each toast and serve.

BEVERAGES

CBD COFFEE *and* TEA

In my research, I've found several ways to make both CBD coffee and tea. You might think that just dumping hot water over hemp would be the way to go—and you could drink that, but, well, it would taste awful. In addition, CBD needs fat, alcohol, or glycerin to be bio-available, so I created these recipes to help you make a great cup of something delicious—and effective.

COFFEE

Using butter instead of cream is a great option; it gives you a "bulletproof"-style coffee.

SERVES 1

1 teaspoon CBD Glycerin Tincture (page 10) or CBD Butter (page 7)
1 tablespoon heavy cream
  CBD Honey (page 21) or other sweetener, to taste
1 cup hot coffee

Add the tincture, cream, and sweetener to taste to the coffee. Stir well to combine.

TEA

You have lots of options with tea: Try adding ½ decarbed hemp and ½ mint or any other herbal tea to your tea ball; you'll find that with the addition of cream and sweetener it's quite good. Have fun and play with this—use different types of tea and adjust the amount of tincture to suit your needs.

SERVES 1

1 cup hot tea (herbal, half unground decarboxylated hemp/half tea, or any blend you like)
1 teaspoon CBD Glycerin Tincture (page 10) or CBD Butter (page 7)
1 tablespoon heavy cream
  CBD Honey (page 21) or sweetener, to taste

Add the tincture, cream, and sweetener to taste to the tea. Stir well to combine.

HOT CHOCOLATE

There are many ways to make CBD hot chocolate, but I want you to have the best. Rich, creamy, and fragrant with cinnamon, this is perfect for cozy nights by the fire. Of course, you can just add glycerin tincture to your cocoa, and that's perfectly fine.

SERVES 4

4 cups whole milk

12 ounces best-quality semisweet chocolate, chopped

¼ cup CBD Flour (page 4)

2 teaspoons cinnamon

1 teaspoon sugar or agave syrup, or to taste

Whipped cream and shaved chocolate, for garnish

In a medium saucepan over medium-low heat, combine the milk, chocolate, flour, cinnamon, and sugar to taste. As it heats, whisk until the chocolate has melted. Reduce the heat to the lowest setting, and cook very gently for 1 hour. Strain through cheesecloth set in a sieve. Garnish with whipped cream and shaved chocolate.

PROTEIN-POWER BREAKFAST SMOOTHIE

I've enjoyed this every day for about a year now—and I'm still not tired of it! It fills me up until lunchtime, too, so that's an added bonus.

SERVES 1

1 cup almond milk, or more to taste

1 frozen banana, chopped

¼ cup frozen blueberries

2 tablespoons peanut butter powder

1 tablespoon psyllium powder

1 teaspoon CBD Glycerin Tincture (page 10) or CBD Alcohol Tincture (page 10; see Note)

Put all the ingredients in a blender and blend well.

note

The CBD tinctures have different tastes and textures, so experiment until you find the type that works best for you.

FRESH FRUIT SMOOTHIE

Use this as a guideline for your smoothies, but go with the fruits that you enjoy and the milk that makes you happy. Most important is enjoying the benefits of CBD at any time of day.

SERVES 2

- 2 cups almond or coconut milk, or more to taste
- 2 frozen peaches, chopped
- 1 cup frozen strawberries
- 1 large banana, frozen and chopped
- ½ cup plain full-fat or 2% Greek yogurt
- 1 cup raw spinach leaves (optional)
- 2 teaspoons CBD Glycerin Tincture (page 10)

Put all of the ingredients in a blender and blend well.

MIMOSAS

Everyone loves Mimosas. But not everyone knows how delicious they can be when made with the right ingredients.

SERVES 6

- 1 bottle (750 ml) good-quality brut prosecco, chilled
- 2 cups fresh orange juice (see Note)
- ¼ cup CBD Alcohol Tincture (page 10), or to taste
  Fresh fruit slices, for garnish

To a large chilled pitcher, add the prosecco, juice, and tincture. Stir lightly to combine. To serve, pour into pretty glasses or flutes and garnish with fruit slices.

note
Orange juice is the classic, but try pomegranate, tangerine, or any other juice you like.

ALMOND JOY

This fun beverage could take the place of dessert: it's rich, creamy, and will make you feel marvelous. The addition of amaretto makes it even more almondy—and joyful. It takes a few hours to infuse the coconut cream, but you can do that ahead of time and keep it in the fridge.

SERVES 2

1 cup coconut cream

3 to 4 grams CBD Flour (page 4)

2 cups almond milk

¼ cup amaretto (optional)

3 tablespoons chocolate syrup

Whipped cream and chocolate shavings, for garnish

To a small saucepan over low heat, add the coconut cream. Tie the hemp in a little square of cheesecloth, and use the string to tie to the handle of the saucepan. Immerse the bundle in the cream and cook for at least 2 hours and up to four (this is the same technique for making CBD Butter or Oil, page 7). The longer you infuse the cream, the more bio-available cannabinoids it will contain.

Remove the bundle and discard. Set aside to cool.

Combine the coconut cream with the remaining ingredients except for the garnishes in a cocktail shaker, and shake with ice. Strain through cheesecloth set into a sieve. Garnish with whipped cream and chocolate shavings.

BLOODY MARY

If you enjoy a Bloody Mary, especially after a tough night, this recipe will truly help you relax. If you just want a delicious cocktail, this does that too! Adjust to suit your taste with more Tabasco, a shrimp garnish, or some CBD alcohol tincture, for example. You get extra points if you salt the rim of the glasses with CBD salt.

SERVES 2

1½ cups V-8 or tomato juice

2 to 3 tablespoons CBD Alcohol Tincture (page 10)

3 to 4 dashes Tabasco sauce

3 to 4 dashes Worcestershire sauce

1 to 2 teaspoons fresh lemon juice

CBD Salt (page 13) and freshly ground black pepper, to taste

2 cups ice cubes

Pickled asparagus, celery sticks, and stuffed olives, for garnish

Place all the ingredients except the garnishes into a cocktail shaker. Shake well, then strain into 2 glasses. Garnish with asparagus, celery, and olives.

SUMMER SPRITZER

Spritzers are perfect for those afternoons when all the chores are done—or you're just done with chores. Almost any fruit is good here, though I've found citrus, especially orange, lemon, and tangerine, are just wonderful. Whatever fruit you use, this is light and refreshing!

SERVES 6

1 bottle (750 ml) vinho verde, chilled

2 cups club soda, chilled

¼ cup CBD Alcohol Tincture (page 10)

Juice and zest of 1 lime

Sliced lime, for garnish

To a large chilled pitcher, add the wine, soda, and tincture. Stir lightly to combine. To serve, pour into pretty glasses or flutes and garnish with lime slices.

RESOURCES

In this book I talk repeatedly about hemp, or *Cannabis ruderalis*, the cannabis plant with less than .03 % THC. You might be wondering, where do I get this hemp? If you don't have access where you live, a great source (and the place I get mine) is LeBlanc CNE. Run by the brilliant Jerry Whiting, LeBlanc is a dependable source for organic, U.S.-grown hemp. Avoid anything not grown in the U.S.; you want a clean, organic product. See leblanccne .com to order.

For information regarding hemp, the legalization movement, or for answers to almost any question you might have, try Leafly. It's a great resource for almost anything cannabis-related. Whether you're looking for a dispensary near you, need a question answered, or are checking up on the latest news, you can find it at leafly.com.

Another good resource is NORML, an organization that educates folks about cannabis and does a lot to advance legalization. With legislation updates and daily news, it's a wonderful reference, and they're helping to get people out of jail and to change laws. Visit NORML.com to learn more.

ACKNOWLEDGMENTS

Our wonderful recipes testers; gratitude to Val McKinley, Jayma Cohn, Ingrid Emerick, Leslie Miller, Tiffany Taing, Emilie Sandoz-Voyer, and Julie (Pie Goddess) Gaunt—you guys are the best!

Jerry Whiting of LeBlanc CNE—thanks for all the delicious hemp.

Everyone at Girl Friday Productions who helped birth this book—thanks, thanks, thanks.

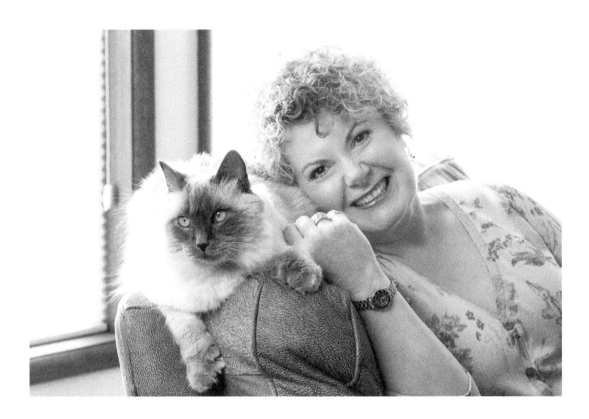

ABOUT *the* AUTHOR

MARY J. WHITE grew up with a spoon in her hand and an apron around her waist, going on to study with Culinary Communion in Seattle. For more than 25 years, she worked in radio, television, and film, appearing on morning and afternoon shows on KUBE, KMPS, KKWF, and KOMO TV, among many others, before transitioning to her second career: teaching people how to cook in hands-on Kitchen Survival classes. In 2011, she began using cannabis to treat hip pain and was astonished at the relief. Since then, she's combined her two loves by teaching classes on how to make infused edibles, topicals, and tinctures.

INDEX

NOTE: Page references in *italics* refer to photos of recipes.